EX LIBRIS

Calista Lee Brown

a handbook of

Yoga

for

modern

living

a handbook of

Yoga

for

modern
living

Eugene S.
Rawls

Photography by
Ed Bollinger

Parker Publishing Company, Inc., West Nyack, N.Y.

Library of Congress Catalog Card Number: 66-14756

PRINTED IN THE UNITED STATES OF AMERICA

38293—B&P

I wish to acknowledge the important contribution to this book made by Eve Diskin, whose experience in the teaching of Yoga enabled her to compile with me the accumulated notes of fifteen years of research in this field.

What Is Yoga?

Yoga, the oldest-known science of self-development, has been found to be the answer to modern man's deepest needs. It solves the problems of health, physical fitness and peace of mind.

Yoga teaches you how to improve and control the condition of *every part*.of your body. It teaches you how to quiet your mind in order to attain real and lasting peace. It is simple and enjoyable.

Yoga is universal. It is for everyone to use regardless of background, age or physical condition. We have taught students from the ages of ten to eighty-one. We have had classes of teenagers, and we have taught Yoga in institutions for senior citizens. Professional athletes have studied with us, and we have had classes composed of handicapped persons.

People use Yoga to overcome their individual problems. Overweight men and women practice Yoga to lose weight. Nervous people use Yoga to calm themselves. Those suffering from fatigue increase their vitality by applying this simple science. Older persons practice Yoga to regain the characteristics of youth.

Americans from all walks of life are turning to Yoga because it has been proven to successfully counteract the occupational aches and pains that every person has. Everyone has some portion of his organism that is below par, stiff, tense or weak. Yoga overcomes these conditions with amazingly little time and effort.

There are two aspects to the science of Yoga, the physical and the mental.

The physical side of Yoga is the science of Hatha Yoga. This consists of cleansing, stretching and breathing techniques.

The cleansing techniques strengthen, purify, massage and stimulate various internal organs of the body. A few of the specific benefits of practicing the Yoga cleansing techniques are:

    a) Normal regularity
    b) Increased resistance to colds
    c) Improved circulation through internal organs

The stretching techniques are called postures. They are a mild scientific stretching of the spinal column and every stretchable part of the body. Some of the benefits you will receive from practicing these wonderful postures are:

    a) Relief from tension
    b) Increased vitality
    c) Youthful limberness and flexibility
    d) A trim and firm figure
    e) Poise, grace and self-confidence
    f) The ability to relax completely

The famous SHOULDER STAND and HEAD STAND belong in the category of postures. These are inversion techniques used for centuries to improve the circulation of blood throughout the entire body. A few of the benefits of practicing these inversion postures are:

    a) Normalized weight (by improving the function of the thyroid gland)
    b) Refreshed brain
    c) Fatigue overcome
    d) Complexion improved
    e) General improvement of blood circulation

Some of the results of practicing the three Yogic breathing techniques as taught in this book are:

    a) Nervous system relaxed
    b) Sleep improved (and, in most cases, insomnia overcome)
    c) Blood purified
    d) Abundant energy gained
    e) Lungs cleansed and strengthened

The mental side of Yoga is the science of Raja Yoga. There are books on Yoga which *talk about* Raja Yoga, but rare indeed are authoritative books giving actual instruction in how to practice these marvelous mental techniques. In this book the science of Raja Yoga is explained in clear everyday terms and you are taught five authentic mental techniques. The results of correctly putting to use the techniques of Raja Yoga are:

a) Calm nerves
b) The overcoming of anxiety, fear, worry, anger and other negative emotions
c) Quieting the mind
d) Experiencing peace

Presidents Eisenhower, Kennedy and Johnson have stressed the urgent need for a national physical fitness program. This is because of their awareness of the declining health of America. Where once we were rated among the top two nations in the world in health, we are now rated below more than half a dozen other countries. Our sickness and disability rate climbs to more alarming heights every year. America needs a *practical, enjoyable* system of physical culture that will keep us at the highest peak of health and that will prevent the negative conditions which come with neglect and incorrect health habits. We need a method of health preservation which can be practiced at home on our own time and with an absolute minimum of expense.

Those who have practiced Yoga for even a few weeks know that only Yoga satisfies these needs. This is because Yoga is *complete* and *perfectly efficient.* Yoga is complete because it reaches and works out *every* part of the human organism, *internal* as well as external. It is perfectly efficient because it always works. If you practice these time-honored techniques correctly, you always receive the benefits claimed for them. It works *automatically.* There is no hit or miss. It is an exact science. If you stretch according to instructions, you *will* become limber. If you become limber in this manner, you *will* free yourself from tension. If you free yourself from tension and know how to be truly relaxed, you *will* gain energy. This is the way it works.

Yoga is non-strenuous. Anyone can begin these mild, delightful postures and movements at once. This book is designed to enable you to sit down *right now* and begin rejuvenating every portion, every organ and gland of your body. All instructions are in the book. There is also a full section on the Yogic viewpoint on food and nutrition. There you will learn in detail the principles and methods of eating for health. Sample menus are included.

All you need to practice Yoga is a private place and a mat or towel to sit upon. By practicing Yoga for twenty minutes a day you are taking one of the wisest and certainly one of the most practical steps of your life. You are taking control of your state of health. No one can live your life for you. Neither can anyone become healthy or attain peace of mind for you. You can only do these things *yourself.* Now, with Yoga, you have the way, the means, of accomplishing every one of the priceless goals stated in this book. By practicing Yoga you are contributing to the health, fulfillment and peace of yourself, your family and society.

The instructions in this book are complete. You will know the how and why of every movement you do. Complete practice schedules are given. Apply yourself to these life-giving techniques as instructed, and you will surely reap the benefits claimed for them.

Contents

Part One

Hatha (Physical) Yoga   I

PRINCIPLES FOR PRACTICING THE PHYSICAL TECHNIQUES
(Continued)

Part Two

Food and Nutrition   117

Part Three

Raja (Mental) Yoga   153

RAJA YOGA: THE SCIENCE OF MIND CONTROL (Continued)

PART ONE
HATHA (PHYSICAL) YOGA

PRINCIPLES FOR PRACTICING THE PHYSICAL TECHNIQUES

1. Practice them according to the time schedules given. Add only the time intervals indicated. Do not be haphazard about the practice of the Yoga postures. Hatha Yoga is an exact science and a delicate art. *Be as methodical and mechanical as possible.* Adhere to the progressive schedule, This is the only way that brings results.

2. Never tug, strain or pull strenuously. You cannot force your body to attain the desired flexibility faster. Forcing will cause your body to resist and will actually slow down or even prevent your progressing. You are not in competition with anyone nor with yourself in the practice of physical Yoga. *Go gently.* Stretch until you reach the point where you "feel" it. Stretch just up to the point where it would start to hurt.

3. *Slow motion is the primary key to physical Yoga.* From the starting position of a posture until you are holding the stretch should take you at least ten seconds and, as you progress, even longer. Count these seconds to yourself in the following manner: "one hundred and one, one hundred and two," etc. Count the holding of your posture in the same precise manner.

4. *Hold the postures* (when you reach your ultimate comfortable stretch) *motionless.* Do not move, squirm or fidget. Do not adjust your body. Your body will do everything if you simply hold it as motionless as a stone in the final position of each posture. Every time you move when holding a posture, you are subtracting from its benefits.

5. *Come out of a posture as slowly as you go into it.* This is an

3

important point where many students fall down. Never collapse out of a posture or come out of it faster than you went in. This negates the good effects for which you performed the technique. Count your way out the same way as you counted your way in.

To summarize:

Increase the time of holding each posture progressively and adhere to your schedule. Count your way, slow motion, into each posture.

Hold the posture without any motion whatever for the prescribed count.

Count your way out of the posture, taking the same amount of time to come out of a stretch as you did to get into it.

STRETCHING POSTURES

THE ALTERNATE LEG PULL

· Restores youthful flexibility
· Relieves tension throughout the spine
· Stretches and develops the legs and back

1. Sit on the floor as in Figure 1, legs extended straight out before you, knees straight, toes and heels together. Your hands are on top of your thighs and your torso is held up as erectly as possible. This is the classic beginning position for many of the concave, or forward bending, postures.

2. Bend your left leg at the knee and bring your left foot up until you can grasp it with both hands. Place the sole of your left foot against (not under) the inside of your right thigh with your left heel as close to your groin as comfort permits. (Figure 2.)

3. Raise both arms in front of you, hands together, at eye level, and, in slow motion, bend forward until you can grasp with your hands the farthest part of your extended right leg that you can reach without discomfort. (This will be your thigh, knee, calf, ankle or foot, depending on your flexibility. It doesn't matter where you reach because with regular, methodical practice you will attain full flexibility in time.) Grip this part of your right leg firmly with your hands.

This part of the technique should have taken you ten full seconds. Count the seconds as you perform it. (Figure 3.)

4. Now, having your grip, bend your elbows outward slowly and gently until you reach the point where you can no longer stretch forward without discomfort. This is the position you will

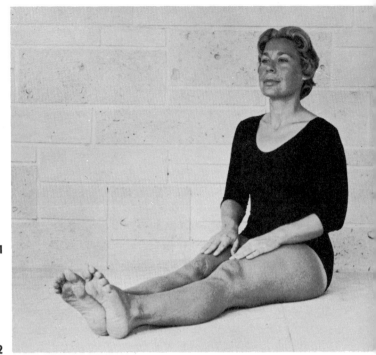

Figure 1

Figure 2

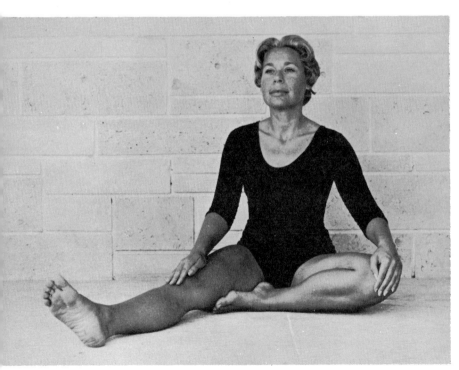

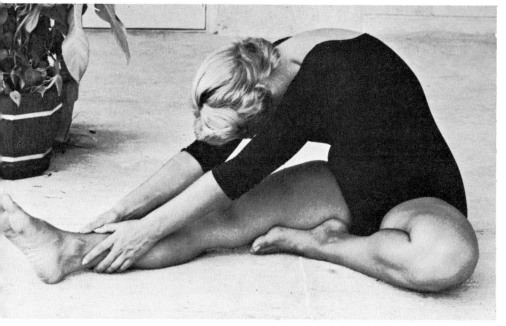

Figure 3

Figure 4

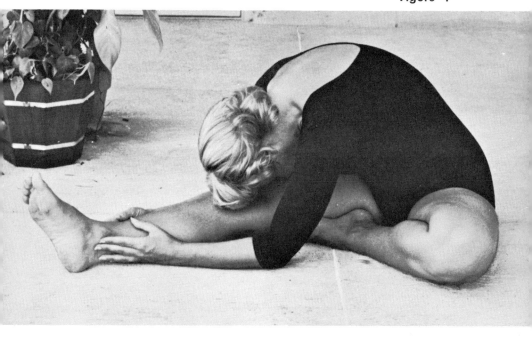

hold, motionless, for the count of ten seconds. Do not move, adjust or fidget. Count the seconds to yourself silently. Keep in mind that your eventual aim is to have your forehead rest upon the knee of your extended leg. (See Figure 4 for this ultimate position.)

Gently is the way. Do not attempt to force your body to stretch farther or faster; it will simply resist and make your progress that much slower. You must enjoy your physical Yoga workout. Let that be one of the criteria for judging the correctness of your practice. In this ALTERNATE LEG PULL for example, you will feel a great stretching in the tendon behind the knee as well as in the back. If this stretching sensation is an actual discomfort, then you are pulling too hard.

5. Coming out of the stretch is an art in itself. First straighten your elbows. Then release your grip on your leg. All this is done in slow motion to a slow, silent count of ten seconds. Next, with the head still down and the neck relaxed, allow your hands to slide up your leg. The bottom of the spine straightens up first and then the middle and finally the cervical vertebrae and the head. At this point you are back in the position shown in Figure 2.

6. The next step is to straighten your left leg out in front of you in a slow, relaxed and composed manner and, bringing your right foot up against the inside of the left thigh, perform the exact movement on the opposite side. This time you will be stretching your left leg and the right side of your back.

Practice Schedule

Do the ALTERNATE LEG PULL three times on each leg (Right, left, right, left, right, left). Take ten seconds to go into the stretch and take ten seconds to come out of it. This is a minimum count to assure correct slowness of motion. But you may feel free to make the time of going into and coming out of the stretch as long as you wish. The slower the better.

But adhere rigidly to the time prescribed for holding each posture.

Hold the ALTERNATE LEG PULL to ten seconds for the first week.

Add five seconds each week to the time of holding the posture. Do this until you are holding the posture for thirty seconds. Then, still increasing the time by five seconds each week, you may do the posture two times on each side. (If you enjoy this posture and wish, you may continue to perform it three times on each side, but two times holding it this number of seconds will produce the desired results.) Continue increasing the seconds at the same rate until you are holding the posture for sixty seconds on each leg.

Benefits

The ALTERNATE LEG PULL stretches every ligament, tendon and muscle of the feet and legs. Atrophied muscles—weak and deteriorated through lack of proper use and manipulation—and other parts are brought to life again by being reached and worked out.

Tension is removed from the many places in which it tends to lodge in the thighs, the calves and the ankles. Tension is relieved throughout the back due to the thorough, scientific and delightful stretching that the back receives.

Nervous tension constricts various parts of the body, making the muscles, tendons and other tissues tight. So long as these tight and constricted areas exist in the body, further tension will accumulate. The scientific stretching of the Yoga postures removes these points of tension and brings in their place genuine relaxation. This is the relaxation and freedom from physical tension that animals give themselves by their natural processes of stretching. Animals retain the intuitive knowledge of how to stretch tension out of their bodies. Man is compelled to learn these ways of nature over again.

True relaxation is not the limp or sleep-inducing kind. True relaxation brings abundant vitality and energy. You will experience this as you practice these postures. First, the posture stretches away the tension at all the points where it has lodged in your body; then, in a little while, you will feel the renewal of energy as the vital force, unobstructed by the draining power of tension, flows through you.

In the ALTERNATE LEG PULL the spine is methodically stretched in a concave (forward) manner so that every vertebra of the spinal column receives an exhilarating and highly therapeutic manipulation. The great spinal nerves which emanate from this column are benefited tremendously by this natural stretching. This posture reduces weight in the abdomen and thighs and tightens up these regions to eliminate flabbiness.

As a by-product of the mechanical performance of this posture, the muscles of the shoulders, arms and upper back tend to become taut and firm.

THE COBRA

- Restores youthful limberness
  - Improves circulation in the kidneys
    - Relieves tension through the entire spine

1. Lie on your stomach on your mat, hands at sides, face on cheek. Go completely limp. (Figure 5.)

It is important to make yourself completely limp before performing each posture and to relax in this limp condition after each stretching posture.

Becoming as completely limp as possible necessitates placing your mind on the various parts of your body and instructing each part in turn to become limp. Start with your feet. Think and feel your feet. Actually tell them to become completely limp. You will feel their response. Then let your attention travel up your body

Figure 5

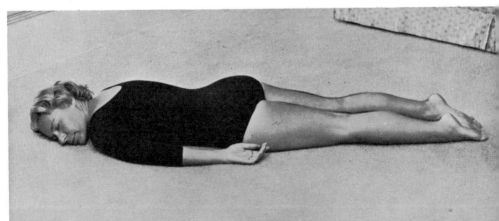

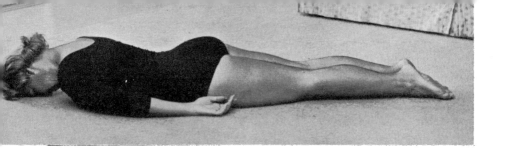

Figure 6

Figure 7

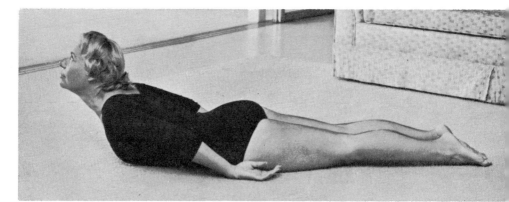

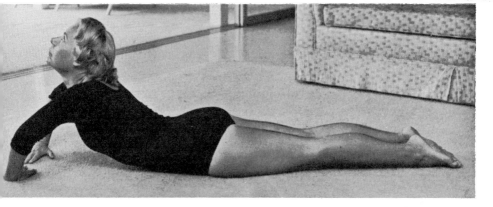

Figure 8

Figure 9

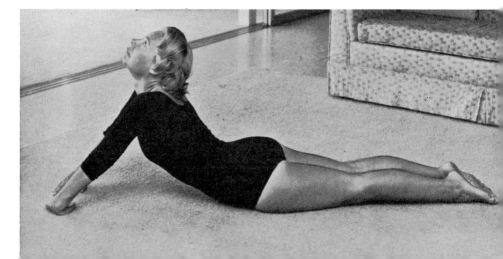

and do the same thing to your calves, thighs, buttocks, pelvis, back, arms, etc., all the way to your scalp. Let this become a habit before and after doing any Yoga posture.

2. Now turn your head so that your forehead rests on the floor. (Figure 6.) In slow motion move your eyes up to the tops of their sockets. When they reach the tops of the sockets, slowly begin moving your head forward until your chin grazes the floor. Move your chin forward until it can go no farther.

3. Using your neck muscles, begin moving your head up until your neck cannot arch back any farther.

4. Using your back muscles, continue raising your head and torso up and back until your back muscles can lift your trunk no farther. (Figure 7.)

Keep your heels together throughout the COBRA posture. This will make it more difficult to bend your spine in this manner, but it is more important to keep the heels together than to gain an extra few inches in the height of your head in the beginning. When the legs spread apart in the COBRA, the pressure is diffused throughout the back. When the heels are together, the pressure is concentrated in a line down the center of the spine, and this is what is desired. Though keeping the heels together may seem to make the stretch more difficult at first, this difficulty is illusory, for in time the spine will stretch in a natural and relaxed manner. Once attaining the complete posture in the COBRA with the heels together, you will have the fullest flexibility that this posture can give, and you will reap the many positive benefits from it.

5. When you can no longer raise your trunk with the use of your back muscles alone, bring your hands *slowly* up from your sides and place them beneath your upper chest near your shoulders, the fingertips of each hand pointing toward each other about six inches apart. (Figure 8.)

Now, using your arms *slightly* for additional support, continue raising your torso up and back as before.

6. When you can go no farther, hold that position motionless

for ten seconds, counting the time silently to yourself. Breathe normally through the nose.

The posture you are attempting to eventually achieve is depicted in Figure 9.

It does not matter if you cannot get into the ultimate position right away. You are not supposed to. If you practice according to instruction, your spine will give, and very shortly you will find yourself able to straighten your arms out.

Never use force nor strenuosity in Yoga. If you simply place your body as far as it will go in these positions, it will stretch by itself and attain the ultimate or complete posture in its own time. It wants to achieve these postures because only by so doing can it feel truly alive, vigorous yet relaxed. So do not practice the COBRA as if it were a pushup. Use no more muscular strength with your arms than necessary.

7. When you have held *your* ultimate position for the pre-scribed count, come down in the same *slow* motion by bending your arms at the elbows.

The slow motion in going up and coming down not only will prevent the straining or pulling of any muscle or ligament but will ensure the complete and thorough stretching and working out of *every vertebra* in your spinal column.

The head is held back as far as possible all the time throughout the COBRA. This is essential to get the complete stretch that is needed. The use of the eyes is the key to correct practice of this technique. Keep them at the top of their sockets throughout the COBRA. The eyes will keep the head properly back. As soon as the eyes lower and look forward you will find the entire stretch is lost. In fact, it has been found instructive for the student to imagine two strings attached to the pupils of the eyes and that these strings are being pulled up and back, compelling the spine to rise in the manner described.

8. When you can support your upper body by the use of your back muscles alone, bring your arms slowly—as if swimming a

slow-motion breast stroke—back to your sides and continue coming down until your chest rests on the floor.

Then lower your head until your chin grazes the floor and finally rests upon the forehead.

Then lower your eyes.

Turn your face on your cheek and make your body, as previously instructed, go limp.

Take twenty seconds to go up into the COBRA. Hold the posture for the prescribed number of seconds. Take twenty seconds to come down.

Half the time of going up (ten seconds) should be done without the use of your arms. The rest of the time of going up (the remaining ten seconds) should be done with the aid of your arms. Apply this timing to coming down as well.

The placement of your hands on the floor acts as an adjuster of the intensity of the stretch. The farther up toward the head they are placed, the easier the stretch. The farther down toward the chest they are placed, the greater the stretch.

If, because of extreme stiffness or other condition, you find the COBRA difficult, you may place your hands on the floor farther up toward your head, under your chin or under your eyes. Later, as you progress, you should place them lower down toward the chest. Actually, the flexibility developed by the COBRA is quick to occur and this paragraph applies only to elderly people or cases of unusual stiffness.

Practice Schedule

Do the COBRA three times at each practice session.

The afternoon or early evening is better than the morning for beginners.

Hold the posture for ten seconds the first week.

Add five seconds a week until you are holding the posture for thirty seconds.

If you practice the techniques in this book regularly, as instructed, you will be amazed and delighted at the results upon your body by the time you are holding the COBRA for thirty seconds.

Benefits

The COBRA, when practiced with sufficient slowness of movement and in correct form, stretches each vertebra of the spine to its normal limit in the convex (backward) direction. This restores to the spinal column its original flexibility. Flexibility is one of the primary characteristics of youth, and when this characteristic is restored to the spine the entire organism not only begins to take on a youthful aspect but increases in many other youthful attributes such as vigor, endurance and a feeling of overall well-being. All the vertebrae and the nerves that emanate from them, from the neck to the base of the spine, are massaged, stimulated and relaxed by this posture.

Certain deformities of the spine have been known to be overcome by this technique. It definitely improves the posture and is especially good in this respect for youngsters in their adolescence who are first encountering postural and other growth problems. All Yoga postures are highly beneficial for young people whose growth processes are not yet complete.

The COBRA provides one of the best illustrations of how the Yoga techniques reach *into* the body and directly work out and affect specific internal organs. Most persons, upon hearing that the Yogi has control over his internal organs, thinks such an ability is some form of superhuman phenomenon. On the contrary, the control that the Yogi has over the internal parts of his organism is based on the most simple, natural and logical physical methods. For example, when you reach the ultimate position in the COBRA where you are holding the posture motionless for a prescribed time (Figure 9), the blood is pressed in a gentle, natural manner out of the kidneys. When you commence lowering your trunk in coming out of the COBRA posture, the blood flows back into the kidneys, thus providing those essential and very delicate organs with a natural internal flushing. This is an extremely healthful thing to do to the kidneys and repays the person who practices it with dividends in health and well-being that cannot be calculated in terms of money.

The COBRA also has positive effects upon the prostate gland

in men and upon the entire sympathetic nervous system. The thyroid gland is mildly stimulated as well.

Weight in the buttocks is reduced by this posture. You will experience the great tightening that must occur in this region when you practice. The muscles of the bust, back and upper chest are developed by this technique, and the muscles of the abdomen are toned and streamlined.

Many persons practice the COBRA immediately upon arriving home after a hard day's work, for they are aware of the COBRA's ability to dispel fatigue.

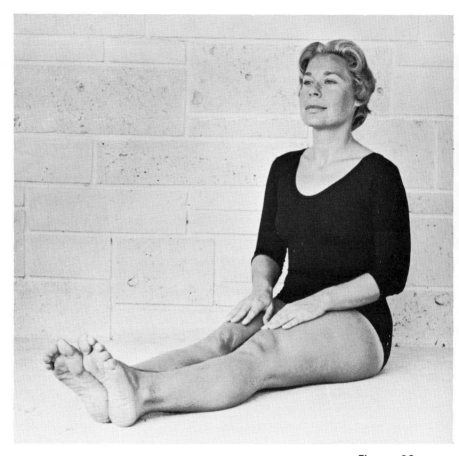

Figure 10

THE TWIST

· Reduces weight in the waist
 · Relieves tension throughout the back and spine
  · Stretches each vertebra of the spinal column

1. Sit on your mat erectly with both legs stretched out in front of you, knees together, heels together. (Figure 10.)

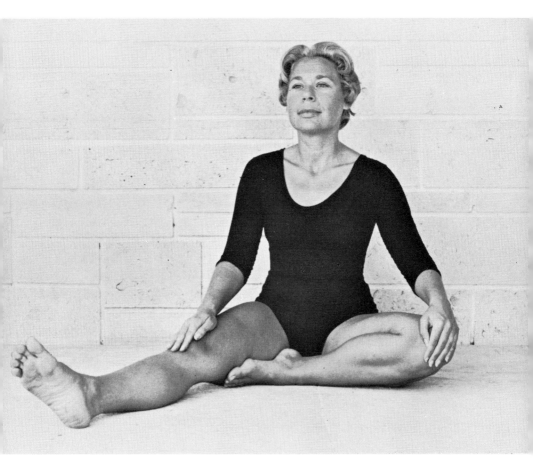

Figure 11

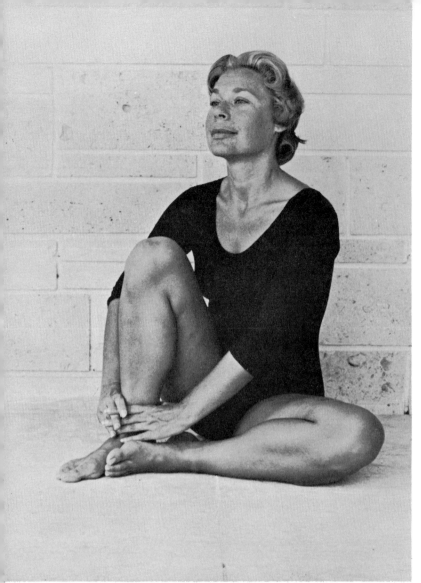

Figure 12

2. Bend your left leg at the knee and bring your left foot toward you so that you can grasp it with your hands.

3. Place the sole of your left foot against the inside of your right thigh, drawing the heel as close to the groin as comfort permits. (Figure 11.)

4. Bend your right leg at the knee and bring your right foot next to or as near as you can to the sole of your left foot. The right

18

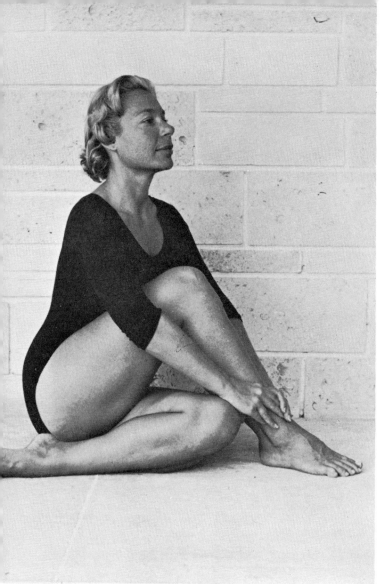

Figure 13

sole, however, must be flat upon the floor and the right knee subsequently high in the air. (Figure 12.)

5. Grasp your right ankle with both hands and lift your right foot over your left knee, placing it firmly on the floor on the left side of your left knee but not too far up toward your left hip. Your right heel should be nearly against your left knee. (Figure 13.)

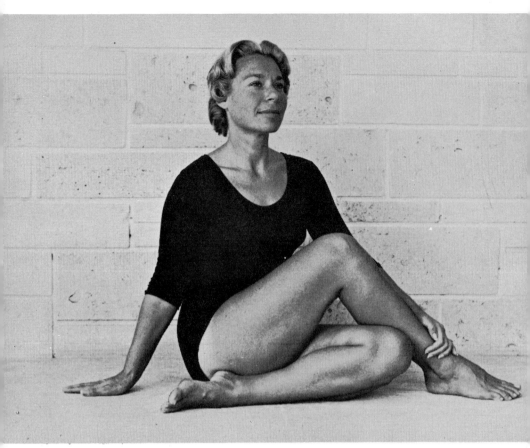

Figure 14

6. Place your right hand on the floor behind you for balance. (Figure 14.)

7. Raise your left arm, the hand at eye level, directly in front of you. Bend this arm all the way at the elbow and hook the elbow over the right knee. (Figure 15.) Now straighten out the left arm so that it extends down the right side of the right leg.

8. Grasp your left knee with your left hand. (If you cannot comfortably grasp the knee, then grasp any part of the shin of the left leg.) You are now in the position depicted in Figure 16.

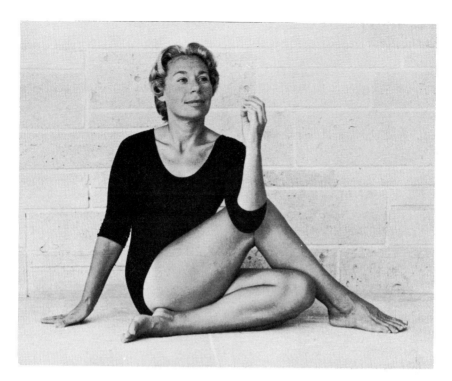

Figure 15

Figure 16

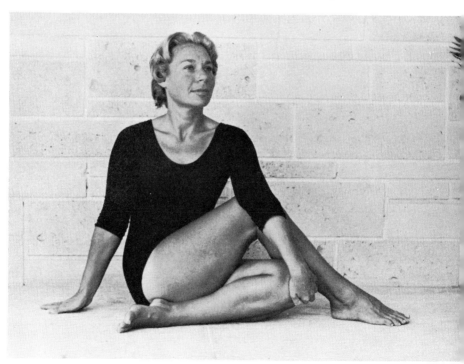

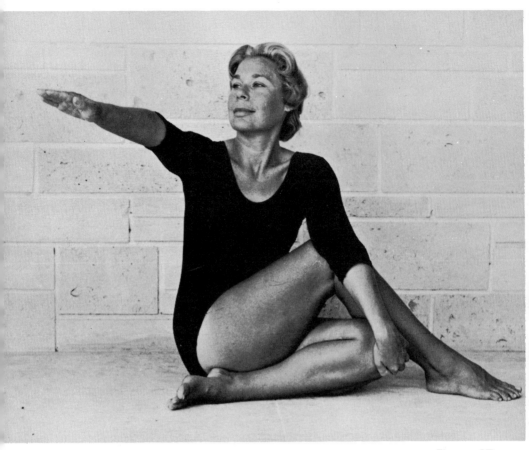

Figure 17

9. Lift your right arm into the air at eye level in front of you. Keep your eyes focused on the back of your right hand. (Figure 17.)

10. *Slowly* move your right hand around to your right, following it with your eyes. (Figure 18.) When you can move your right arm no farther around, bend it at the elbow and allow the hand to drop (always in the same slow motion) and reach around behind you until it clasps the left side of your waist. For the correct basic position of the right hand, see Figure 19.

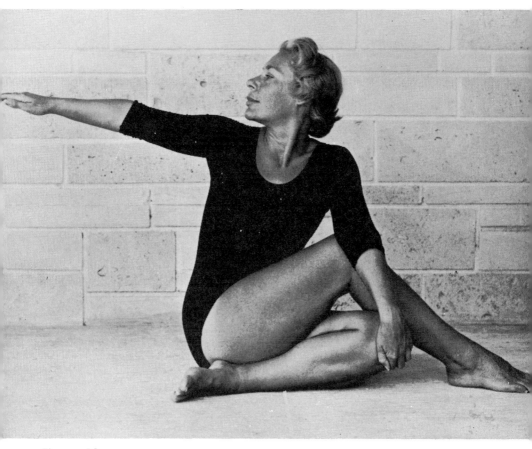

Figure 18

11. You are now in the position depicted in Figure 20. Your eyes are as far to the right in the sockets as they can go. The eyes are directing the TWIST. The neck is stretched to its maximum rightward, although, as always, very gently.

Due to the slowness of the movements involved in placing your body in this posture, the spinal column has been twisted into this spiral stretch very gently and systematically.

Hold this posture for ten seconds, counting to yourself in the prescribed manner.

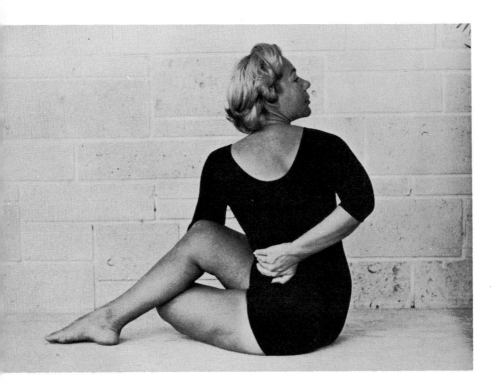

Figure 19

Figure 20

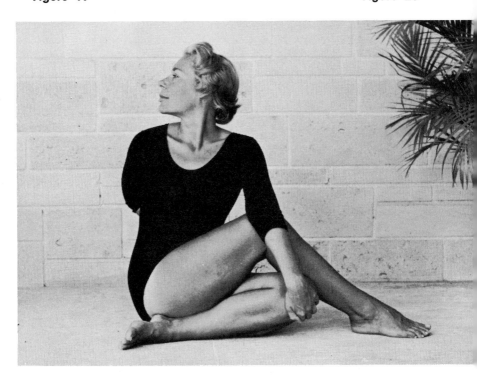

12. To come out of the TWIST, bring your right hand down from the back where it holds your waist and place it on the floor behind you for support.

Now gently release your left hand from its hold on your left knee. Grasp your right ankle with both hands. Lift your right leg back over your left leg and set your foot on the floor beside your left foot. Extend your right leg straight out in front of you. Then extend your left leg the same way so that you are once again sitting in the original starting position.

From this point you will perform the TWIST on the other side, twisting the spine to the left, by going through the same steps starting with the right leg bending at the knee, placing the right sole against the upper inside of the left leg at the knee, etc.

Note: The TWIST is the most complicated of all the techniques you will learn in this book. It is extremely ingenious. Note Figure 16. The left arm is locking the right leg in place. The right leg in turn locks the lumbar (lower) region of the spine forward. Against this stationary lower segment of your spine, you methodically twist the rest of your spinal column in a spiral or corkscrew manner.

Note the right foot in Figure 14. Moving this foot nearer to the body or farther away from it makes that leg an adjusting lever. The nearer to the body the foot of the leg that has crossed over the other leg, the greater and more intense the stretch. The farther away from the body you move the foot that has crossed over the opposite leg, the less intense will be the stretch. Persons suffering from extreme overweight who may find the TWIST difficult to get into, may extend the leg that has crossed over the opposite leg as far out as they wish. Little by little, as the weight normalizes itself through the practice of these postures, the extended foot may be brought back closer and closer to the body.

Many people will find that a problem of keeping the balance as well as a shortness of breath will exist when first attempting the TWIST. The body quickly accommodates itself to these postures, and those symptoms soon disappear. Pay no attention to them. All Yoga techniques are completely natural, and the body loves to do them. With regular, enjoyable practice, stiffness will be overcome. Stiffness is the primary characteristic of old age. When you regain your normal original flexibility, you will feel marvelously youthful and alive.

Practice Schedule

Do the TWIST three times on each side (Right, left, right, left, right, left). Hold the posture motionless for ten seconds. Add five seconds each week to the holding time. Build up your time at this rate until you are holding the TWIST for thirty seconds.

Benefits

In Yoga we emphasize improving and maintaining the health of the spinal column and all the nerves connected with it by means of gentle, methodical and natural stretching. In order to do this we bend and stretch the spine convexly—backward—as in the COBRA and the FISH, and now in a spiral or corkscrew manner by means of the TWIST.

All the impulses that come from the brain to the body and return from the body to the brain must pass through the spinal cord, which is the great nerve of the body. This nerve is ensheathed in the middle of the bones of the spinal column. The great nerves that run from the spinal cord to all parts of the body come out of each vertebra of that spinal column. Like any other part of the human body, this vital region will deteriorate if it is not used properly.

The tongue is not exercised by talking. The feet are not exercised by walking. Similarly, the spinal column is not exercised by the everyday movements which it makes. Indeed, it is not even partially exercised by its everyday movements. Sitting in chairs and automobiles the way we do compresses the spine and puts it so far out of its correct normal condition that people by the hundreds of thousands each year have to go to chiropractors and osteopaths to have the position of the vertebrae adjusted.

The health of the spine and the great nerves that emanate from it depends upon correct scientific manipulation. That is one of the functions of Hatha Yoga.

The Yoga system of spinal adjustment and conditioning is a form of chiropractic self-applied. This strongly applies to the TWIST. Here the spinal column is taken like a chain, the top link and the bottom link of which are being turned in opposite directions. Each link, or in reality each vertebra, is being gently and scientifically twisted to its natural limit, relieving the tension of the entire muscular system of the back connected with this movement and strengthening the nerves themselves. The spine becomes flexible once again in the spiral manner, and the entire nervous system directly connected with the spinal column is stimulated and toned.

The TWIST improves poor posture and also has been known to correct certain spinal deformities.

Flabbiness and excess weight are removed from the waist by means of the technique.

The great sciatic nerve in the region of the hip joint is benefited, the thighs tend to become more taut and firm, and the hip joint itself is limbered and worked out.

There is considerable effect from the TWIST upon the internal organs. Mainly, it stimulates and improves the circulation of blood in the abdomen and kidneys.

You will find the muscles of the shoulders are developed and toned by this technique.

THE LION

· Removes wrinkles
· Improves circulation in the throat and face
· Reconditions sagging face and neck muscles

The LION posture is a technique that appeals very strongly to women. It deals with the elimination and prevention of sagging and wrinkling of the face.

Here is how the LION posture is practiced.

1. Sit in the Japanese sitting position, on your knees, with the tops of your toes extended behind you on the floor. The weight of your buttocks is on your heels. (Figures 21 and 22.)

2. Place the palms of your hands upon your knees. Straighten your elbows. Push your chest forward and stretch your back up-

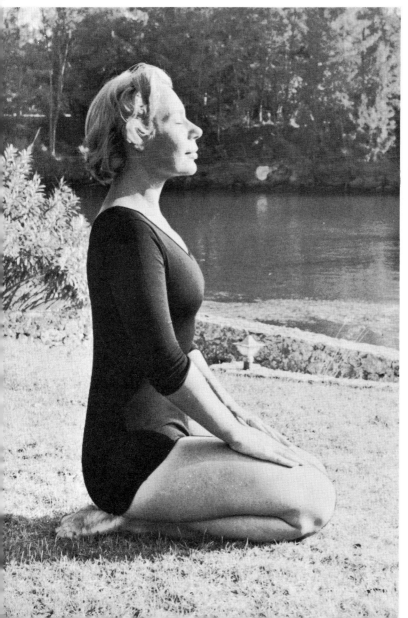

Figure 21

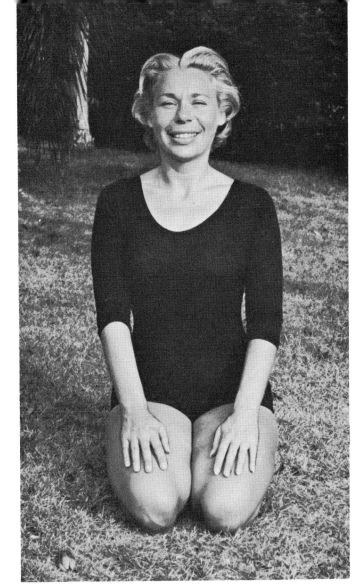

Figure 22

ward as erectly as you can without taking your weight off your heels.

3. In this position, perform the following movements:
   a) Spread your fingers as wide apart as you can.
   b) Open your mouth as wide as you can.
   c) Extend your tongue as far out of your mouth as possible as if attempting to touch your chin with the tip of it.
   d) Open your eyes as wide as you can.

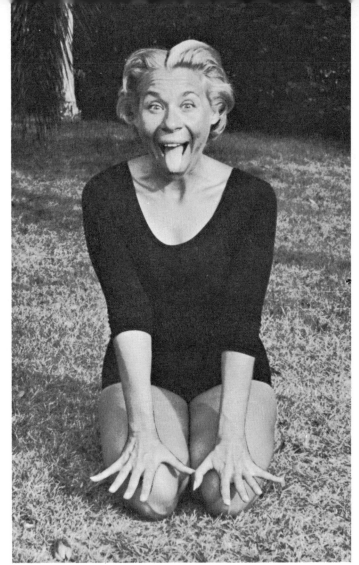

Figure 23

4. Hold this posture for ten seconds. (Figure 23.)

5. Draw your tongue back into your mouth slowly. Return to the beginning position shown in Figure 21.

6. Sit for several moments enjoying the great relief from tension that you will experience throughout your face. Then repeat the stretching movements.

Practice Schedule

The LION posture may be performed at any time of the day that is convenient for you when you feel the need to relieve the accumulated tension in the region of the face.

Begin by holding your tongue out for ten seconds. Add five seconds each week until you are holding your tongue out for thirty seconds each time. Do this three times, that is, three extensions of the tongue at each sitting.

For best results practice it three times each day, although one session each day (three stretches) will suffice.

Benefits

Talking and eating do not exercise the tongue and throat any more than sitting exercises the buttocks. Only a *methodical, scientific* manipulation of that region can benefit the health of it. The LION posture is the ultimate natural movement for affecting positively the face, tongue and throat. The results are very definite.

By stretching your face in this manner, you will eliminate many wrinkles which have appeared around the corners of your mouth and around the corners of your eyes. If such wrinkles in your skin have not appeared, this posture will be instrumental in preventing them. This does not apply to the wrinkles or lines in the forehead.

The wrinkling we have referred to—crow's feet, etc.—is mainly the result of poor circulation in skin of that area. The region above the heart is (unless you practice the Yogi inversion techniques such as the SHOULDER STAND or the HEAD STAND) suffering throughout your life from improper blood circulation. This prevents minute impurities from being thoroughly eliminated from the skin of the face. By stretching the skin as in the LION posture, in time these wrinkles which are caused by poor circulation will begin to disappear.

Stretching the skin of the face in this manner tones the skin and muscles deeply. This result cannot be duplicated by any external means except perhaps extreme and usually painful chemical or surgical methods.

The effect of the LION posture upon the skin of the face is cumulative and in time tends to become permanent.

When people reach their middle years, the greater majority suffer from the unsightly and uncomfortable condition of sagging necks. This is a demoralizing as well as an unhealthy and unnecessary condition. It is simply the loss of the natural resiliency and tone of the muscles beneath the jaw and in front of the neck.

The LION posture restores the natural healthy condition of these muscles, and once more the skin of this area is drawn taut and youthful in appearance.

The inside of the throat is never reached in a correct therapeutic manner. Once again Yoga reaches *inside* your body to increase the health and well-being of your internal parts.

The stretching of the root of the tongue improves the voice by its relaxing and strengthening affect upon the region directly around and connected to the vocal cords.

The salivary glands inside the mouth are affected in a positive manner, improving their functioning, improving the circulation of the tissues surrounding them and stimulating the glands themselves.

The LION posture improves the circulation of blood in the face even more strongly when it is practiced in conjunction with —directly after—the SHOULDER STAND and/or the HEAD STAND.

Tension is removed from the muscles of the face, neck and throat by practicing this technique. You will immediately feel this relief from tension. This effect becomes so delightful that many persons practice the LION for this reason alone.

The name of this posture is derived from the fierce expression of the face and also from the extension of the fingers while performing it. The LION extends his claws just before springing. Many of the Yoga techniques are named in such a poetic fashion. But there is benefit even in the extending of the fingers. This stretching also serves to relieve and eliminate the tension that has accumulated in the hands.

By sitting throughout this posture in the Japanese sitting position you gain the extra benefit of stretching out and thus relieving tension in the feet.

THE PLOUGH

• Improves the complexion
  • Helps reduce weight
    • Stimulates and massages internal organs

The PLOUGH begins in much the same manner as the SHOULDER STAND.

1. Lie on your back. Go completely limp. (Figure 24.)

2. Stiffen your legs, tighten your abdominal muscles and raise your legs to a 90 degree angle from the floor. (Figures 25, 26 and 27.)

Figure 24

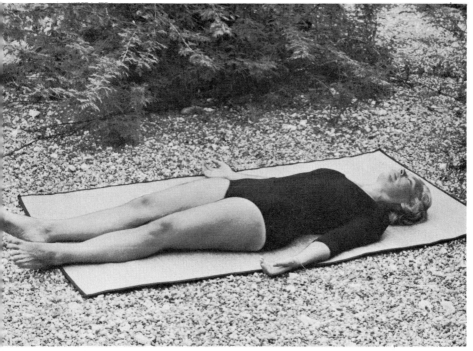

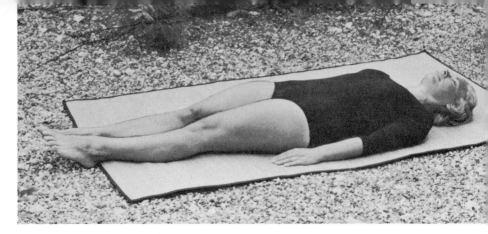

Figure 25

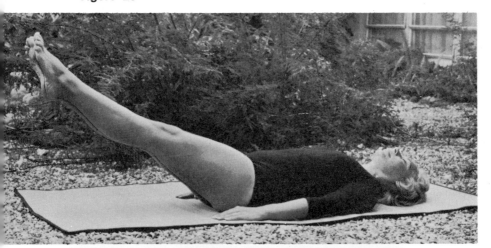

Figure 26

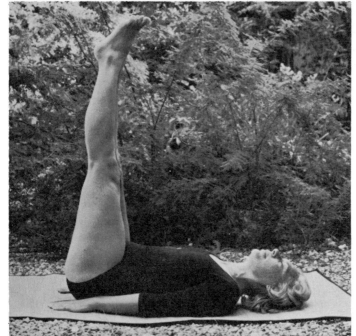

Figure 27

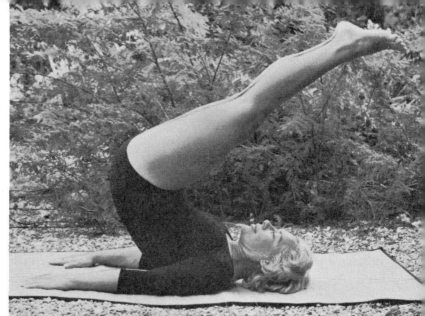

Figure 28

Figure 29

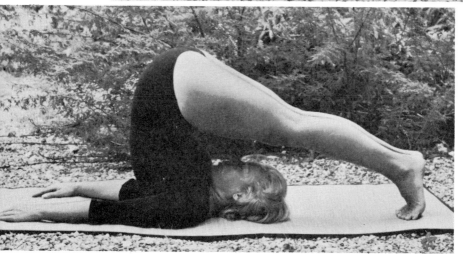

3. Aided by pressure applied by your hands against the floor, at your sides, raise your buttocks and lower back off the floor so that your legs rise over your body, feet moving toward your head. (Figure 28.)

Unlike the SHOULDER STAND, however, the body will not straighten up into the air.

Bring your feet back over your head until the toes touch the floor behind your head. (Figure 29.) Hold this position motionless for five seconds.

All movement is done as slowly as possible.

4. Now slowly bring the arms up and clasp them on the top of your head. (Figures 30 and 31.)

You will find as you practice that this second position permits a greater stretch to the spine and your toes will reach an inch or more farther in back of your head.

Hold this position motionless for five seconds.

5. To come out of the PLOUGH, bring your arms down from your head and place your palms down on the floor in front of you for support. (Figure 29.)

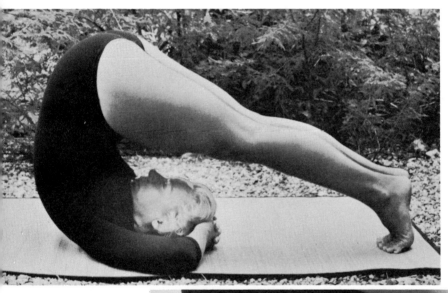

Figure 30

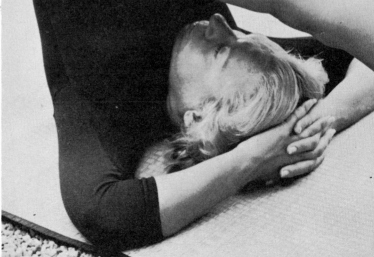

Figure 31

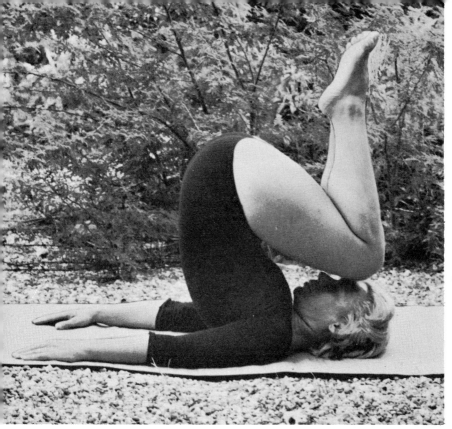

Figure 32

6. Bend your legs at the knees, bringing your knees as close as you can to your face. (Figure 32.)

7. Now, arching your head back so it does not lose contact with the floor, roll *slowly* forward like a ball until you are once again reclining full length on your back. (Figures 33 and 33A.)

8. Go completely limp and rest for at least thirty seconds.

If, upon first attempting the PLOUGH, you cannot assume the first position (Figure 29.), you should practice the PLOUGH posture for the prescribed number of seconds at the farthest position that you can comfortably maintain. An example would be Figure 28.

You will find that the spine tends to stretch quickly into the PLOUGH posture and that day by day the stiff and tense muscles, tendons and vertebrae give another inch and then another inch until the toes reach the floor in back of the head as in Figure 29.

37

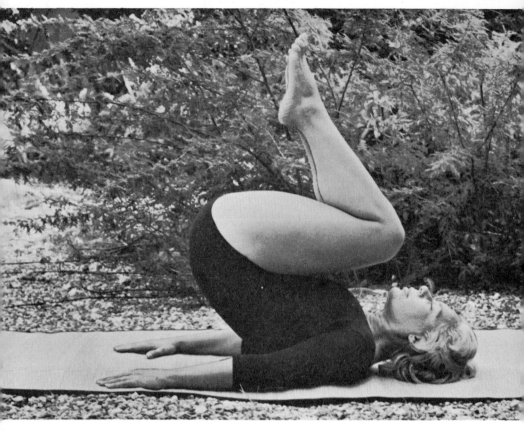

Figure 33   Figure 33A

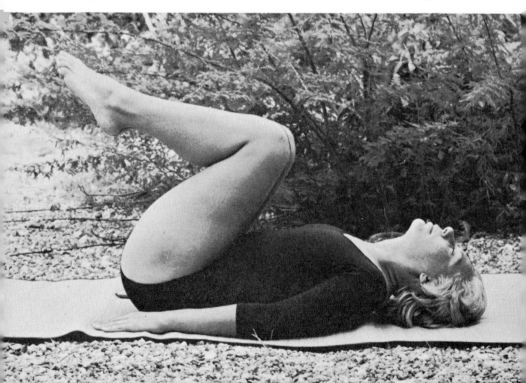

Practice Schedule

The PLOUGH should be practiced in conjunction with the ALTERNATE LEG PULL, either before it or after it, whichever your body seems to prefer. This will form a concave or forward-stretching group in the same way that the COBRA and the FISH form a convex or backward-stretching group.

Start holding each position of the posture for five seconds.

Add five seconds a week to each position of the PLOUGH until you are holding each position for thirty seconds, or, in other words, holding the entire PLOUGH posture for sixty seconds.

Benefits

The PLOUGH is an intense and thorough stretching of the spinal column, especially the middle region and the neck. The raising and lowering of the legs tighten and develop the abdominal muscles, making that region firm and trim. The muscles of the neck are strengthened as well as stretched, and the stretching of the back muscles in this posture relieves tension throughout the back. Youthful elasticity is regained.

The habits of our daily life compress and stiffen our spinal columns. This column of separate bones wants very much to stretch out to its normal and relaxed condition once again. The PLOUGH is a concave posture which gives the spine the incentive to do just that.

Here you will see the relation of energy or vitality to relaxation. A person with tense points in his or her body cannot be relaxed even if he lies down limply and very often is unrested even after a night's sleep. Nor can a tense person ever have his full vitality. Tension drains vitality. Energy is lost from a tense person much as water is lost through holes along a leaky water hose. The tense points in the body correspond to the holes in the hose in this simple analogy. Conversely, true relaxation—or absence of tension —brings energy.

The PLOUGH is a splendid way of learning this by experience. For it invariably happens that, once even the slightest degree of flexibility commences to occur in this posture, the student will feel extremely relaxed, even drowsy, while in the PLOUGH. But, if he takes sufficient rest after coming correctly out of the PLOUGH, in a few minutes he will feel the energy begin to surge through him. This is the real natural vitality of man, not the false energy brought about by artificial stimulants such as caffein or benzedrine, and, as such, functions slowly and smoothly in the body and lasts a long time.

The PLOUGH is weight-reducing for the hips, thighs and abdomen.

It has a massaging effect upon the heart, lungs, liver and spleen, and serves to stimulate the reproductive glands and organs.

To a great degree the PLOUGH is an inverted posture. It is good for the complexion of the face and has a noticeable effect in relieving headaches and soothing—through improved circulation and stretched position—the eyes and other organs of the head when they are feeling the effects of tension and strain.

THE LOCUST

· Increases strength of the groin and lower back
· Stimulates internal glands and organs
· Reduces weight in the hips and thighs

Our most vital muscles and glands are weakened and deteriorated by the inactivity of our bodies in this machine age. Here is a time-honored Yogic technique which strengthens the muscles of the groin area and lower back and has a wonderful therapeutic effect upon the sexual glands and organs. It is the only Yoga technique which involves any strenuosity. You must put a little effort into the LOCUST, but remember that the rewards are well worth it. This posture is only held for a very few seconds at a

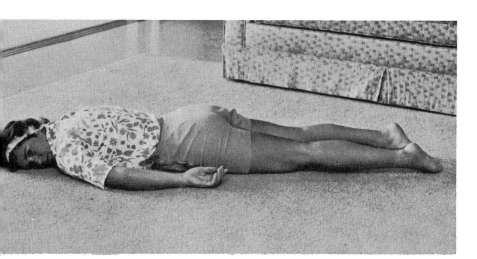

Figure 34

time. The other deeply beneficial effects are explained under Benefits.

1. Lie face down on your mat. Allow your body to become completely limp. (Figure 34.)

2. Bring your heels and toes together, the toes extending outward.

3. Clench your hands into fists and place your fists *thumbs down* directly at your sides.

4. Place your chin firmly on the floor with the pressure nearer to the lower lip than on the point of the chin. You are now in the position shown in Figure 35.

5. Inhale half a lungful of air, enough to use to brace yourself with but not enough to break the firm balance of the preparatory position that you are now in.

6. Holding the breath *in* and using the strength of your abdominal muscles, raise your legs off the floor as high as you can. Try not to bend your knees. Press down against the floor with your fists as you raise your legs.

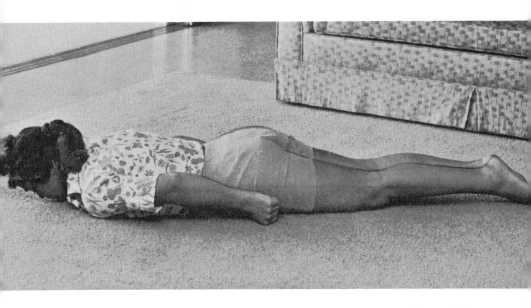

Figure 35   Figure 36

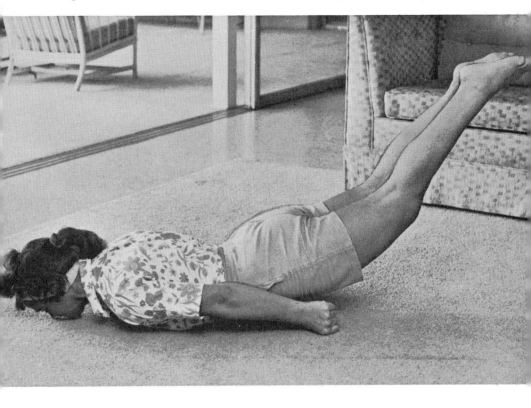

7. Hold your legs up in the air for five seconds. You are now in the posture shown in Figure 36.

8. Lower your legs as *slowly* as you can. Do not collapse out of this posture.

9. When your legs once again rest on the floor, release the air from your lungs in a controlled manner.

10. Allow your body to become completely limp and rest this way until you are ready to perform the LOCUST for the second time.

Practice Schedule

Do the LOCUST three times.

Begin by holding the posture, your legs in the air as high as you can hold them steadily, for five seconds.

Add *one second* a week. This may seem like a very little, but many years of teaching experience has proved to me that if a beginning student attempts to raise the time duration of this posture at a faster rate than this, he will hinder himself from progressing in this wonderful therapeutic technique. As always, the slower you move and the slower and more methodically you make yourself progress in this refined science, the more perfect will your progress and development be.

Continue to add one second a week to the LOCUST until you are holding it for ten seconds. If you find that you enjoy the feeling of strength and stimulation that comes with perfecting the LOCUST, you may continue increasing your time at the same rate.

Benefits

The LOCUST is a natural, wholesome stimulant to the sexual glands and organs, kidneys, intestines and liver. The lifting movement that brings about the stimulation and improved circulation in these vital organs also strengthens and develops the abdomen, lower back, thigh and buttock muscles. The arm and shoulder muscles are also developed and toned by practicing this technique. The vertebrae of the lower spine, with emphasis upon the sacroiliac region, are adjusted by the practice of the Locust posture. Due to the way in which pressure is concentrated toward the triangle formed by the two fists and the chin, the thyroid gland is stimulated and the heart experiences a beneficial massage. The Locust helps eliminate excess weight in the hips and thighs.

THE HALF LOCUST

Those of you who, due to age, excessive weight or other reasons, simply cannot get started with the Locust, should practice the HALF Locust.

The HALF Locust is identical in every way to the Locust with the one exception that instead of raising both legs simultaneously off the floor, you only raise one at a time. (Figures 37 and 37A.)

The leg that remains on the floor presses against the floor and further aids in lifting the other one. You will find the HALF Locust much easier than the Locust. Begin holding the HALF Locust for five seconds and add five seconds a week until you are holding each leg in the air for thirty seconds. Then begin practicing the Locust in place of the HALF Locust.

THE LEG AND BACK STRETCH

1. Sit in the basic Yoga beginning position. (Figure 38.) Keep your legs straight and your feet together.

2. *Slowly* raise your arms straight out in front of you, thumbs together and the backs of your hands at eye level. (Figure 39.)

3. Lean back a few inches. Make sure your back is straight and your chest is as far up and out as possible. This will stretch your rib cage and your waist and will make certain that you receive the greatest stretching effect when you go into the posture. (Figure 40.)

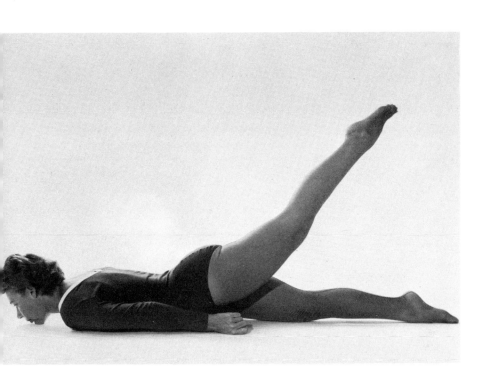

Figure 37   Figure 37A

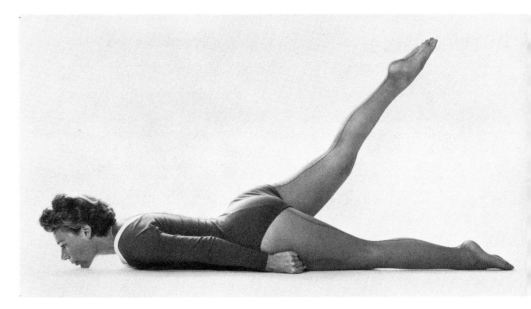

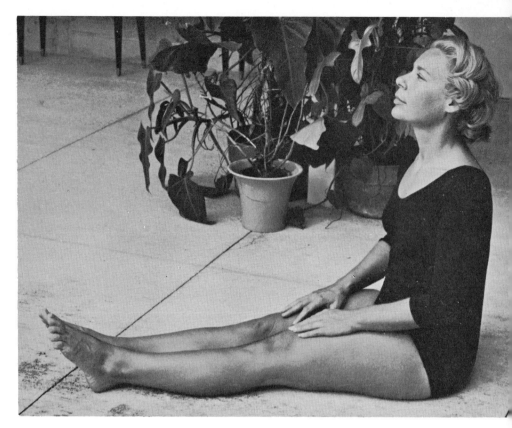

Figure 38   Figure 39

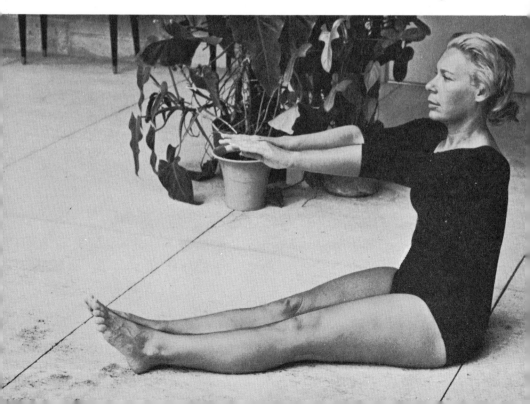

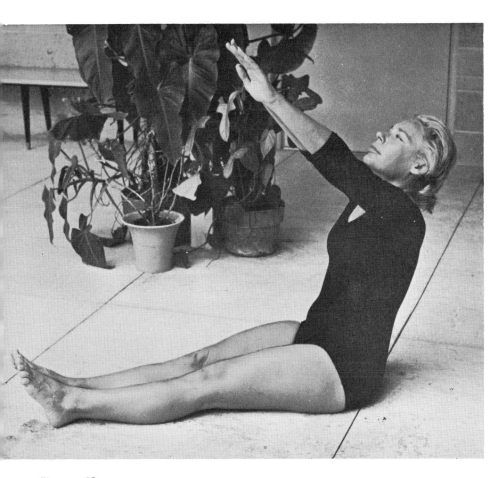

Figure 40

4. Come slowly forward until you grasp the farthermost part of your legs that comfort permits. (Figure 41.) It doesn't matter if it is your feet, ankles, calfs, knees or thighs.

5. Now bend your elbows slightly and, aiming your head at your knees, apply a *gentle* pull until you feel that you are experiencing just the right stretch for you.

Do not strain or exert any undue force. The postures must always feel comfortable and the stretching sensation must always be mild and enjoyable. If it actually "hurts" then you are doing

47

it too hard. Remember, if you simply place your body into these
postures as far as it can pleasantly go, your body will do all the
rest of the work for you.

You should take at least ten seconds from the starting position
until you begin to hold the stretch.

6. Hold the position *without moving* for the prescribed amount
of time. In this posture start out by holding it for ten seconds.

Do not fidget, adjust your position or move about. And above
all, don't rock up and down in order to stretch a little more. This
will retard your progress. See Figure 42 for the ultimate position.

7. Come out of the LEG AND BACK STRETCH by reversing the
steps by which you went into it.

First straighten your arms. Then straighten your back, starting
from the base of your spine and progressing upward until your
neck becomes erect. Let your hands slide up your legs so that
when you have straightened up out of the posture, you are once
again in the starting position shown in Figure 38.

Always come out of a posture as slowly as you go into it.

Practice Schedule

Do the LEG AND BACK STRETCH three times.
Hold the posture for ten seconds.
Add five seconds each week to this time until you are holding
the posture for thirty seconds.

At this point you may repeat the LEG AND BACK STRETCH only
twice. Build your time up at the same rate until you are holding
the posture for sixty seconds.

Benefits

The LEG AND BACK STRETCH is the ultimate concave stretching
posture. Complete flexibility of the back and legs is restored by
this technique.

It stretches and works out every vertebra of your entire spinal
column. The great nerves which emanate from your spinal column

Figure 41

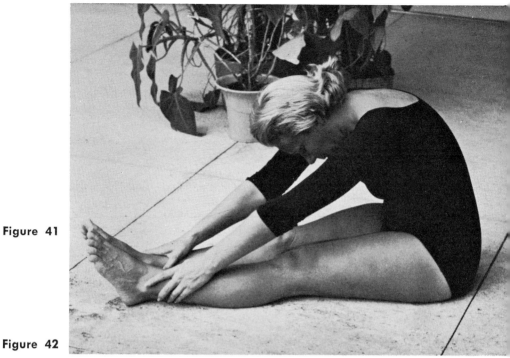

Figure 42

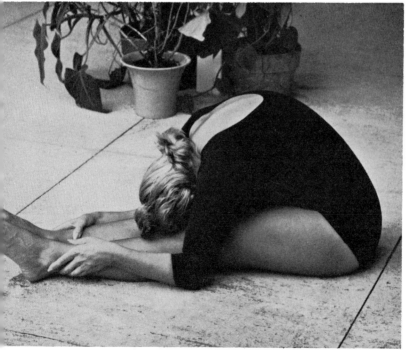

and go to *every* part of your body are strengthened, toned and relaxed by this posture. Accumulated tension is eliminated throughout the back and spine.

Because the points of tension are stretched away in this manner, your natural reservoir of energy is tapped and made available to you. Tension drains vitality. Eliminate tension, and vitality flows freely through your organism. By regularly practicing the stretching postures you will experience this for yourself.

The LEG AND BACK STRETCH strengthens the muscles of the shoulders, upper back and arms.

The great tendons of the back of the legs are stretched out to their original flexible condition by this posture. These are among the first parts of the body to stiffen. This stiffening and tightening up of these areas robs you of energy and of the natural endurance that you should have. This Yoga technique will restore the full use of your legs.

It is highly weight-reducing for the waist, abdomen and hips.

It adjusts—as do all the stretching postures—the vertebrae of the spine, but in this instance with special emphasis on the lower vertebrae and the sacroiliac.

This posture has a definite effect on the internal organs. It massages and stimulates the colon, reproductive organs, kidneys, liver and stomach.

Do not look for overnight attainment of the ultimate flexibility in this particular technique. You have spent the greater part of your life in becoming stiff, tense and tight in the areas worked out by the LEG AND BACK STRETCH. This posture will not "give" as quickly as the others. But you will receive the full benefits as soon as you begin practicing it, and you will feel the wonderful relief from tension and the delightful long-lasting surge of vitality that it brings. Everyone who practices according to the instructions will attain the complete posture in time.

THE BOW

1. Lie face down on your mat. As with all Yoga postures, pre-

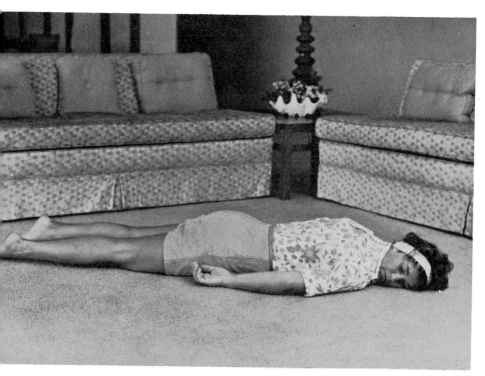

Figure 43

cede the posture with a brief period of complete limpness. (Figure 43.)

2. Turn your head so that your forehead rests upon the floor and bring your toes and heels together.

3. Bend your legs at the knees and, reaching back with your hands, grasp hold of your ankles or feet. (Figure 44.)

4. Once having this hold, inhale a complete breath.

5. As soon as the breath is inhaled, with a moderately fast motion—not the same strict slow motion as in nearly all the stretching techniques—raise your head and trunk off the floor as in the Cobra and at the same time, aided by your arms, lift your legs off the floor as far as you can.

Use the strength of your arms to help in the raising of your legs.

51

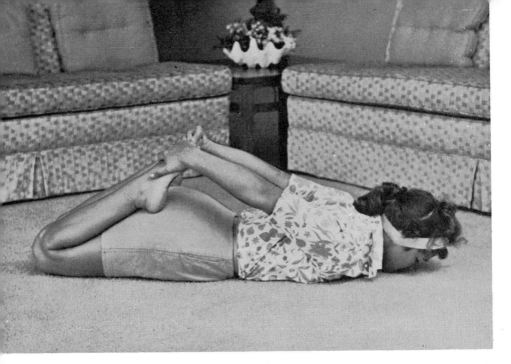

Figure 44   Figure 45

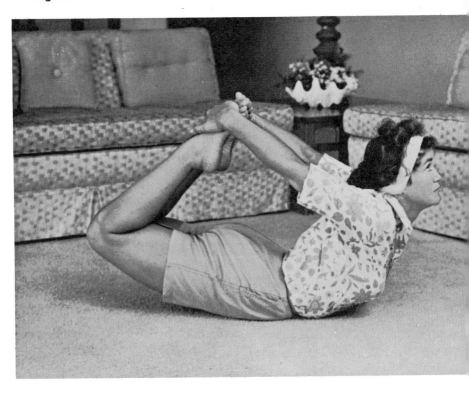

Your neck is bent as far back as possible. You retain your breath throughout the holding of this posture. (Figure 45.)

6. The body is now bent like an archer's bow.

After holding this posture for the required length of time, lower your trunk and head to the floor. Then lower your thighs to the floor.

Exhale your breath in a controlled manner.

7. Release your ankles (or feet) and allow your legs to straighten into the original reclining position.

8. Rest limply.

Practice Schedule

Perform the Bow posture three times.

Hold the final position—legs and trunk in the air—for five seconds the first week.

Add one second a week until you are holding the posture for fifteen seconds. Do not progress faster than this.

Benefits

The Bow posture strengthens and develops the entire back, adjusting the large vertebrae of the lower spinal column—lumbar and sacroiliac—and greatly improving the posture.

It strengthens the arm and shoulder muscles as well as the muscles of the abdomen. Strengthening the abdominal wall, it encourages the visceral organs to remain firmly in their proper place—high and held in firmly.

The chest cavity and bust are developed by this technique.

The Bow helps reduce excess weight in the abdomen, thighs and hips.

It also reaches within the organism and affects positively the internal organs. The thyroid gland, kidneys and pancreas are the main organs stimulated by this posture.

THE FISH

· Relaxes and strengthens the nervous system
· Relieves tension throughout the body
· Keeps the feet strong and healthy

Actually, this is a modified FISH posture. The complete FISH posture is done with the legs in the FULL LOTUS position. It is more important for a beginner to receive the benefits of the convex stretching of the spine which this posture so efficiently imparts.

1. Sit in the traditional Japanese sitting position, as shown in Figure 21.

2. Slowly inch your hands back along the floor until they are situated behind you at shoulder width and supporting you, as in Figure 46.

3. Keeping your buttocks on your heels, let your head fall limply back, in slow motion, and bring your abdomen up and forward, bending your spine in a convex manner. (Figure 47.)

4. Hold this posture for ten seconds motionless, breathing normally and quietly.

This is the preparatory position for assuming the FISH posture. It should be practiced every day. It will limber your spine so that you can place your body into the next position. Do not attempt the next position until you are holding this first posture for forty-five seconds. Increase your time by adding five seconds each week to the duration of this technique. Then experiment gently day by day to see if you have gained the elasticity needed to go into the following position.

5. Slowly and gently, feeling your way into the position inch by inch, bring your elbows down on the floor behind you with your hands grasping your ankles. Go only as far as you can each day, holding the position when you reach your limit of comfort.

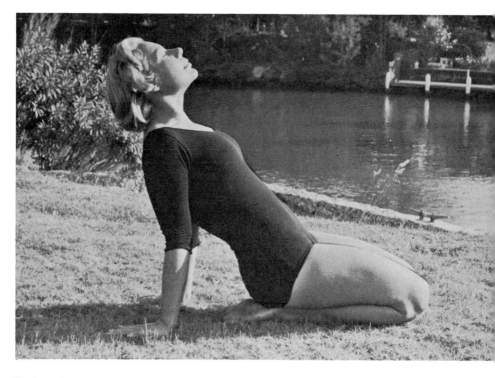

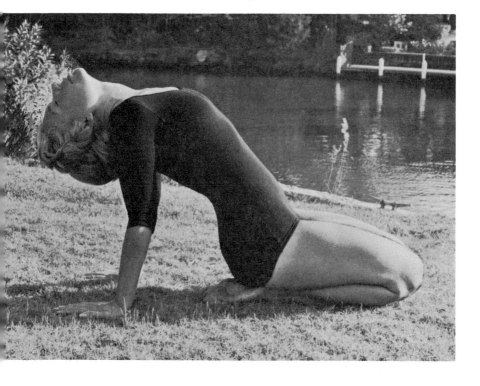

Figure 46   Figure 47

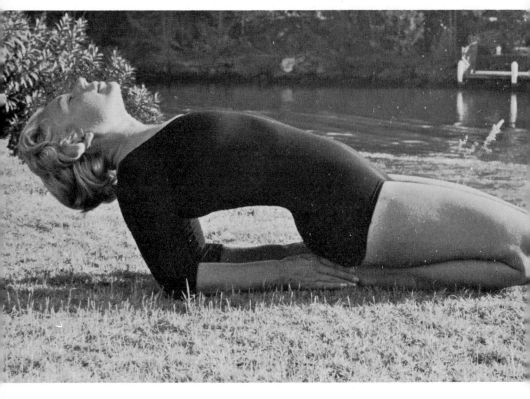

Figure 48   Figure 49

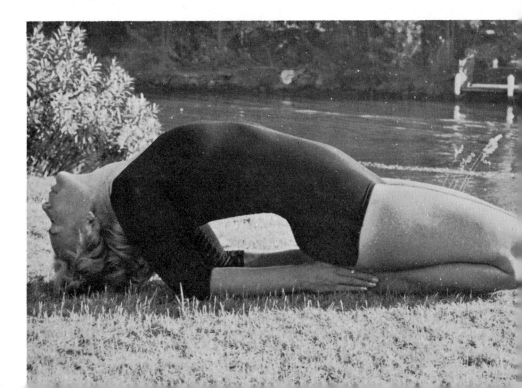

A pleasant, moderate stretching sensation is all that is required. (Figure 48.) Your head drops back limply, your knees are held together throughout this technique, and you hold this position for ten seconds motionless.

6. In time, as your body, with slow and methodical care on your part, adapts itself to this second stage of the FISH, you may, very slowly, work yourself into the final position.

Gently allow your head to come lower, a fraction of an inch more at each practice session, until the top of your head rests on the floor. (Figure 49.)

7. Hold this posture for ten seconds.

8. Come out of the FISH posture very slowly and carefully. Never lurch out of it or roll quickly from one side to another. Come up in stages, as slowly and methodically as you went down.

Do not push yourself to enter the second stage of the FISH until you are quite relaxed and comfortable in the first. When you think your spine has regained enough elasticity to be ready to go into the next stage, experiment by gently feeling your way down an inch or so at a time.

There is never any hurry in Yoga. Hurrying, or pushing yourself in any way in this science, will definitely slow or even stop your progress. You cannot force development in Yoga. You will learn the deeper significance of slowness in the mental, or Raja Yoga section.

Practice Schedule

This posture should be practiced as the last of the convex series (COBRA, LOCUST, BOW, FISH.)

Hold the posture shown in Figure 47 for ten seconds the first week. Add five seconds each week to this holding time. Do this three times.

When you have built your time up in this manner until you are holding this posture for forty-five seconds, then you may commence lowering yourself back onto your elbows.

When you begin to practice the phase of the FISH posture shown in Figure 48, begin again at ten seconds. Add five seconds each week to the retention of this posture until you build up to thirty seconds. Be sure never to progress faster than this. You have been repeating this technique three times.

When you reach thirty seconds, you may repeat the posture only twice if you wish.

When you reach forty-five seconds you may perform this posture only once.

Build your time up to sixty seconds.

As you practice, your head will automatically lower itself from the position in Figure 48 to the complete posture. (Figure 49.)

Allow this stretching to happen in your body's own slow, natural way.

Benefits

The first positive effect of the FISH posture will be the rejuvenation of one of the most abused parts of the human body, the feet. The average person considers the foot to be a sort of insensitive brute portion of the body which is made, like a hoof, to withstand any kind of treatment. But witness the countless millions of dollars spent each year on treatment by chiropodists and on patent cures for foot trouble. Witness also the scores of bodily miseries which result indirectly from misuse of those appendages. First we encase the feet in suffocating and constricting leather contrivances or, in the case of women, devices which crush and twist the feet and throw the entire spinal column out of balance. Then we neglect to systematically and correctly care for or "exercise" them. The result is that the toes have become nearly vestigal appendages and the feet themselves, besides becoming susceptible to numerous ailments, are points of great accumulation of tension.

From the beginning of the FISH—where you are simply in the traditional Japanese sitting position—to the final posture, your feet are stretched out in the most natural and therapeutic manner possible. All the tension is removed from these areas, the nerves there are strengthened and the use of your feet and ankles is increased. The Yogis maintain that the steady practice of this posture will significantly aid in preventing arthritis from settling in the feet.

Tension is likewise removed from the great muscles and tendons of the front of the thighs. The tendons of the knees are stretched back into their normal condition.

The spinal column is stretched convexly (as in the COBRA) with the emphasis being placed upon the lower portion, especially the sacroiliac.

The muscles of the abdomen are toned, and much tension is removed from the groin area.

There is a general positive effect upon the glandular system from this stretch, once the final stage is reached and can be rested in with the body relaxed.

THE SIMPLE POSTURE

This is the everyday cross-legged posture with which we are all familiar.

Figure 50 demonstrates this SIMPLE POSTURE. Its main use in Yoga is to help those persons who are not yet able to assume the HALF LOTUS or FULL LOTUS sitting postures. Through constant use of the SIMPLE POSTURE, your legs will become prepared for the practice of the HALF LOTUS.

If you cannot sit in the HALF LOTUS, sit in the SIMPLE POSTURE as much as you possibly can each day. It is highly advisable to

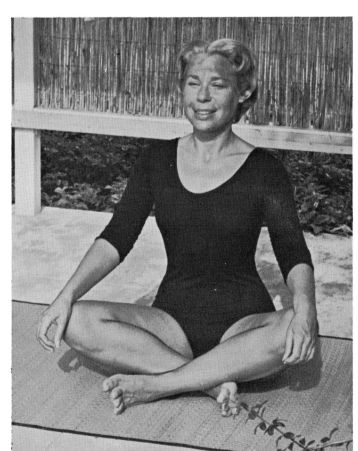

Figure 50

61

begin the practice of sitting on the floor at home at every occasion —to read, to watch television, etc.

The everyday sitting position that we employ in the Western world is extremely unhealthy for the internal organs, for the spine, for the nervous system, for the legs and for the mind. This may seem like an extreme statement, but it is quite true.

Chair-sitting is far from comfortable. After only a few minutes of sitting in a chair you are invariably obliged to move your legs. Indeed, if you will observe, people are constantly fidgeting and shifting their legs about while sitting. This is actually the fault of the position. The nerves are irritated by prolonged chair-sitting. The circulation of blood through the legs is impaired. The condition of the muscles, joints and tendons is eventually deteriorated by the customary sitting position that we use every day. We will go into more detail as to the positive benefits of sitting in the Yogic manner in the section on the benefits of these particular postures.

THE HALF LOTUS

1. Sit on your mat with both legs extended straight out in front of you, feet together.

2. Bend your left leg at the knee until you can grasp your left foot with both hands. Place the sole of your left foot against the inside of your right thigh with the heel drawn as close to the groin as possible. If you can, insert the toes of your left foot *slightly* under your right thigh. (Figure 51.)

3. Bend your right leg at the knee until you can grasp your right foot with both hands. Lift your right foot and place it, sole upward, upon the cleft where the left thigh and calf come together. The right heel should be as close as comfort permits to the area just above the reproductive organs and should be resting lightly against the abdomen at that point.

4. Place the wrist of each hand upon each corresponding knee. Rest your arms lightly and in a relaxed manner in that position. Sit erectly. (Figure 52.)

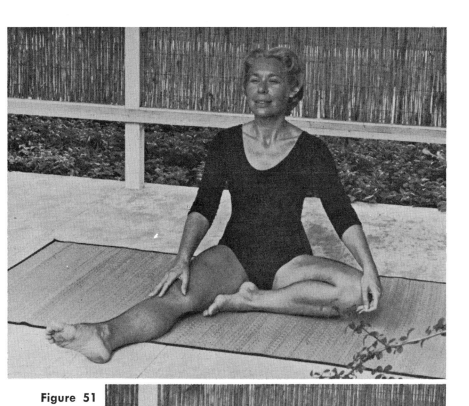

Figure 51

Figure 52

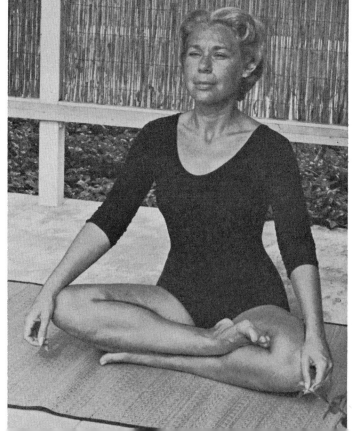

Most persons will find in the beginning that the right knee is in the air and cannot rest in the correct relaxed fashion upon the floor. *Do not force, push or "work out" the upraised knee under any circumstances.* The sheer weight of the leg itself will work out the stiff ankle and hip joints and stretch in a natural manner the stiff tendons of the inner thigh which prevent the leg from assuming its natural, correct sitting position. Your leg will lower itself in time. If you simply sit in the HALF LOTUS as often as you can each day, you will see the upraised leg lower itself a little more each time until it rests upon or very close to the floor. Manipulating the stiff or upraised leg with your hands or placing undue pressure upon it to accelerate the regaining of its natural elasticity will slow the process and expose you to the possibility of unnecessarily straining a part of that leg.

These are all *natural* positions for the body to be in, and it wants very much to be in them, for only then can it feel truly comfortable and relaxed. You have but to place your body in these postures as far as it can comfortably go and *it* will do all the rest by itself, in its own time stretching out and attaining the ultimate stage of relaxed elasticity.

THE FULL LOTUS

The FULL LOTUS is an advanced posture and is quite difficult for the greater majority of people to get into. This is because of our lifelong unnatural sitting habits as well as the excessive accumulation of calcium and other mineral deposits in the knee and other joints of the legs.

Regular practice of the HALF LOTUS will prepare your legs for assuming the FULL LOTUS.

Success in meditation—mental Yoga techniques for attaining peace of mind—is *not* dependent upon being able to sit in the FULL LOTUS.

1. Sit in the classic beginning position just as you began the HALF LOTUS.

2. Bend your left leg at the knee until you can grasp your left

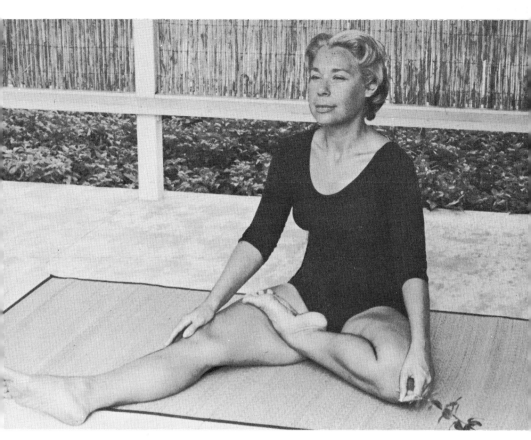

Figure 53

foot with your hands. Lift your left foot and place it, sole upward, upon the top of your right thigh. Bring your left heel in as close as you can to your abdominal wall. (Figure 53.)

3. Bend your right leg at the knee until you can grasp it with your hands. Lift your right foot up and over your left calf and place your right foot, sole upward, upon the top of your left thigh. Bring your right heel as close as you can to your abdominal wall.

Once again rest your wrists lightly on each corresponding knee and sit erectly. (Figure 54.)

Practice Schedule

Sit in whichever of these postures is most comfortable for you on every occasion you can during the day. Reverse your legs,

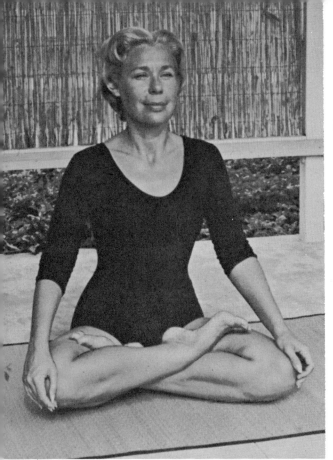

Figure 54

placing the one that was on the top on the bottom, so that both legs are worked out and developed equally.

Definitely employ these sitting postures when practicing any of the meditation—Raja Yoga—techniques and any of the physical techniques that require sitting.

You should practice the HALF LOTUS as soon as you are limber enough to get into it.

Benefits

The practice of the HALF LOTUS posture will loosen your knee joints and ankles. The loosening of the knee joint comes about, to a great degree, through breaking down the excessive mineral deposits which have accumulated in that area.

Once this process begins to take place, your blood begins to circulate more correctly through that joint. Most people suffering with arthritis who have studied Yoga with me have informed me that as the HALF LOTUS commenced to loosen their knees and ankles, the pains of their arthritic condition correspondingly diminished.

The Yogis maintain that such conditions as arthritis cannot occur in a part of the body that has proper circulation and that, further, the practice of the LOTUS POSTURES, especially when combined with the other postures, will serve, to a very great degree, to prevent these afflictions.

At the same time that the LOTUS POSTURES loosen the ankle and knee joints, they work out and stretch the tight and insufficiently used tendons that run along the inside of the thigh from the knee to the groin. By restoring the original elasticity of these tendons—muscles and ligaments as well—you will find that you nearly double the use and endurance of your legs. Where you could have walked or stood for two hours before, after stretching out and reconditioning these inner thigh tendons you will be able to use your legs for twice that length of time before feeling fatigue.

Sitting with your legs stretched delightfully (and it is a delightful sensation once these parts begin to give and stretch out), your entire pelvic region is strengthened and rejuvenated. The seldom-used muscles of the groin area are strengthened and benefited, and many parts of the pelvic girdle, from the groin to the hip joints and around through the muscles of the kidney region, are toned.

When you thus loosen and stretch your legs so that you can once again sit in man's natural sitting position, a very strange and wonderful phenomenon begins to take place. Due to the positive alteration of the blood circulation in the legs—which constitute a large percentage of the bulk of your entire body—and due to the relief from tension in this entire area from the stretching process, the metabolism is affected in such a way that the tempo of the breathing tends to slow down. When you study the breathing techniques taught in this book, you will become acquainted with the enormous implications of our breathing. But here it will suffice to say that sitting in the LOTUS POSTURE slows and lengthens the breathing and that slowing the breathing in conjunction with the particular stretching of the legs that the LOTUSES impart, along with other factors, *produces a general calming of the entire nervous system.*

As the breath slows down and becomes less erratic, so does the mind become quieter, less restless and less subject to all forms of agitation. This is a mechanical process which happens automatically.

We are all accustomed to the term "psychosomatic," which designates that condition where the mind affects the body— usually enough to show visible symptoms. But it is easy to forget the more obvious truth, that the body has a direct effect upon the mind. Calm your body and you calm your mind. The breath is, eventually, the main factor in the body's control of the mind.

This is why the Yogis for thousands of years have employed the HALF LOTUS, or natural sitting position of man, as their way of sitting. Besides the benefits to the physical organism, there is this quieting effect upon the breath, nerves and mind.

Moreover, there is the matter of simple comfort. Our western sitting position is extremely uncomfortable. Once your limbs begin to stretch into and accommodate themselves to the LOTUS POSTURES, you will for the first time in your life find out what comfort in sitting is. In the ultimate positions of the LOTUSES, one actually forgets about one's limbs. No movement is necessary.

The LOTUS POSTURES do not come quickly to most people. Have patience. Always remember that you do not have to be in the ultimate position of a Yoga posture in order to obtain its profound benefits. Every time you do it, no matter where you are on the road toward complete flexibility, you are gaining the fullest benefit to your organism.

I have used the expression the LOTUSES, grouping the FULL LOTUS and the HALF LOTUS together. This is because all these remarkable properties and values to your body and mind apply to both of them. The FULL LOTUS simply is a more intense application of them to your organism.

THE SHOULDER STAND

· Normalizes weight
 · Improves circulation
  · Nourishes and refreshes the brain

1. Lie on your back, with your hands at your sides, palms up. Go completely limp.

2. Stiffen your legs and tighten your abdominal muscles. Place

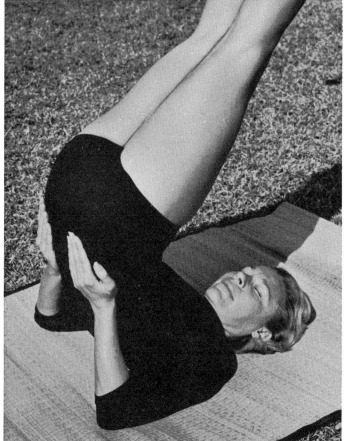

Figure 55

69

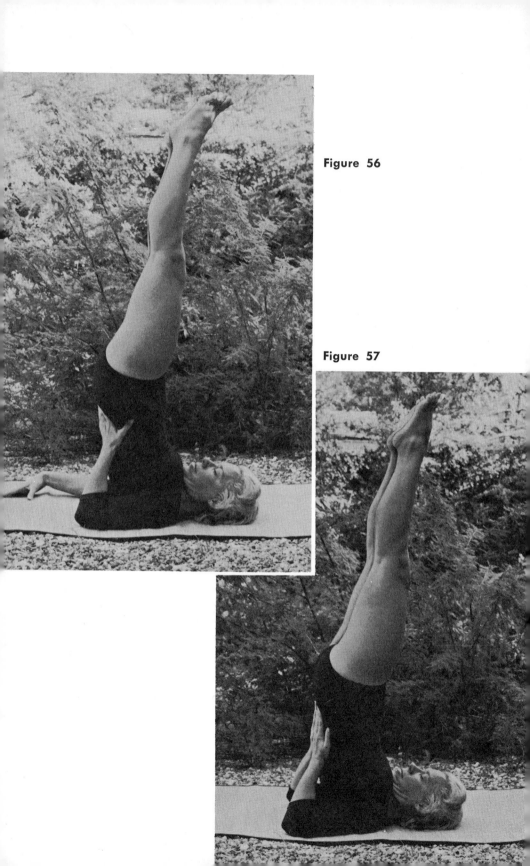

Figure 56

Figure 57

your palms downward against the floor. Raise your legs slowly heels together, until they form a 90 degree angle to the floor. Aid the raising of your legs by pressing downward against the floor with the palms of your hands. (See Figure 27.)

3. By continuing to press against the floor with your hands, raise your lower back off the floor until your legs are in the air over your body as in Figure 28.

If because of overweight or muscular weakness you cannot raise your lower back off the floor, you may rock or manipulate your body and get into the position of Figure 28 by whatever means necessary. (Figure 55.)

4. Bend your arms at the elbows and brace your hands against the kidney region of your lower back, thus aiding in the support of your upraised legs and trunk.

If you have a balance problem, you may place one hand in position first, bracing your body with it, and then place the other hand in position for support. (Figure 56.)

5. Now continue raising your body up until you are in the complete posture as shown in Figure 57.

If you cannot attain this complete posture, simply go as far as you can comfortably. The body adapts to the SHOULDER STAND quickly, and in a few days or weeks you will find that you can comfortably remain for the required time in the complete posture.

In the completed SHOULDER STAND most of your body will be able to remain quite relaxed, only the biceps of your arms having some tension. This work on the part of the arms is correct. The upper chest or jugular notch will be pressed against your chin.

Sometimes, especially in the beginning, the head and face will feel flushed and throbbing. This is good, for it indicates an accelerated circulation of blood through that area. After a little while you will cease to feel it so obviously. This increased circulation is one of the desired qualities of the SHOULDER STAND.

6. Hold the SHOULDER STAND motionless for three minutes. Three minutes is the *minimum* time for holding the SHOULDER STAND. You do not get half the benefit by holding it for half the

time. It does not work that way. It takes three minutes for the effect to take place.

7. Come out of the SHOULDER STAND in the following manner:
Bend your legs at the knees. Bring your knees *slowly* down as close to your face as you can. (Figure 57A.)

Place one hand palm down against the floor and brace yourself with it. Once braced, place your other hand on the floor. (Figure 57B.).

Now, supporting yourself with your hands against the floor, and with your body rolled up like a ball, roll *slowly* forward until your lower back once again rests on the floor.

Straighten your legs up into the air and lower them as slowly as you can (this will develop your abdominal muscles, making them firm and strong) until your heels rest on the floor.

Rest completely limp for at least one minute.

It is essential never to come out of an inverted posture fast. Never allow yourself to roll out of the SHOULDER STAND immediately into a sitting position.

You must keep complete control of the process of coming out of the SHOULDER STAND. To do this, it is necessary to practice the following technique: Once you are braced with your hands on the floor and are ready to roll out, simply make sure that the back of your head does not leave the floor. No matter how far back you have to arch your neck, keep your head in contact with the floor. This will enable you to keep control over the rolling out, and you will find that you can come down in the correct slow motion and not roll forward into a sitting position.

The SHOULDER STAND should be practiced in the afternoon or early evening. It has tremendous ability to recuperate the body from the effects of the day-long pull of gravity.

Practicing the SHOULDER STAND as the first of your Yoga techniques is usually desirable because of its positive effect upon the circulation of blood through your entire body.

It should be practiced every day, one time, holding it for three minutes. You may increase this time to as much as ten minutes

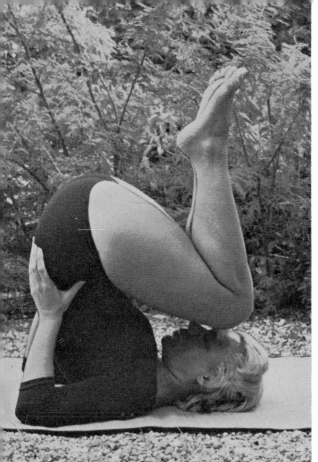

Figure 57A

Figure 57B

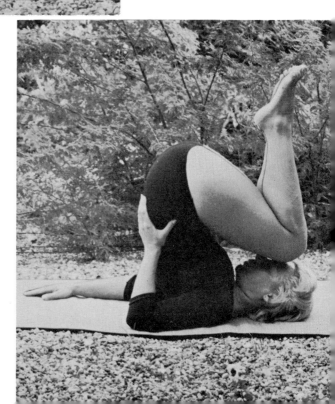

if you do so in a methodical manner by adding thirty seconds a week.

Benefits

The SHOULDER STAND is one of the greatest blessings to man. Everyone should practice it daily for the promotion of health. The effects upon the body of the SHOULDER STAND could be a course in themselves. We shall briefly outline the main ones here.

Keeping in mind the final inverted posture, we shall start with the legs and work down toward the head describing the results of practicing the SHOULDER STAND three minutes every day.

Gravity is constantly pulling on us every second of the day, and most of the day we are on our feet. The average person certainly does not have the occasion to have his feet above his head in the course of his usual daily life. The heart has to push the blood quite forcefully to circulate it back up the legs to the upper body. This, plus the force of gravity, plus the customary use of our legs, causes great pressure upon the walls of the blood vessels of the legs. In time, in a certain percentage of people, this pressure distends the walls of the veins, causing a painful and pathological condition which can eventually develop into varicose veins.

Through the years it has been found that the SHOULDER STAND, practiced each day after the day's work is done, and held for a minimum of three minutes, has a very positive effect upon that condition. In the inverted position there is less pressure on the walls of the blood vessels of the legs. This enables them to contract and recover from the continual strain. In time they regain their natural condition.

The internal organs and glands are also subject to the pull of gravity all day long. They hang in position as well as lean upon one another in one particular way all that time. When the body is inverted, they hang and lean, as it were, upside-down. Parts of them are relieved of pressure and other parts are stimulated by different kinds of contact with other organs. These internal organs —including nearly all the visceral organs—are immensely relaxed by this position as well as nourished by the improved circulation of blood.

The sexual organs and glands are benefited by the SHOULDER STAND. In men, a regeneration of the sexual glands occurs. In women, the effect is tremendously therapeutic, all of the inner reproductive glands and organs falling back gently into their natural place. This posture is very beneficial for women suffering from misplacement of the uterus and is being more and more prescribed by doctors for women to practice after childbirth. In men, this posture has a positive effect upon the prostate gland.

There is also a positive effect upon hemorrhoids if the SHOULDER STAND (in conjunction with other techniques) is practiced with greater intensity, that is with the time of holding the posture built up beyond the normal moderate limits given in this book.

Note. At this point we reiterate that we are not in any way prescribing these techniques medicinally. Only your physician is qualified to diagnose and prescribe for a pathological condition. We are simply stating the facts that have been observed and tested by modern scientific standards and have worked for countless numbers of people now and through centuries past.

Due to the stimulation of the visceral organs, those which have the function of eliminating waste—kidneys, liver—are improved in that functioning. This is as much due to the movements involved in going up into the posture and coming down out of it as it is in the improved circulation through the inverted organs.

One of the main values of this technique is its ability to normalize and redistribute body weight. Many persons in our country, knowing the danger to health and longevity of excess poundage, have taken instructions in physical Yoga for this reason alone. The way this works is by the effect of the inverted position upon the thyroid gland.

The thyroid gland is to a great extent the controller of weight in the human body. Through years of misuse—by wrong diet and other improper treatment of the body—the thyroid gland becomes sluggish and can no longer perform the function that keeps the body weight normal. External means—pills, even surgery—cannot make the thyroid gland function normally. Such means can only adjust it temporarily or temporarily relieve an extremely pathological condition. The thyroid gland must be stimulated to correct activity internally, and only you can do that.

By standing in the SHOULDER STAND for the prescribed time, with your chin tucked against the notch formed by the top of your breastbone and the insides of your collar bone, the blood flow soon concentrates at the location of the thyroid gland. The thyroid gland is then massaged and stimulated by the increased circulation of blood through it. It commences once again to secrete in the correct quantity and manner those chemicals which in turn regulate body weight.

Nourishing and stimulating an internal organ through increasing the circulation of the body's own blood through it is the most natural therapeutic thing that one can do to a body part. There is no such thing as the thyroid gland being overstimulated by the SHOULDER STAND. This cannot happen. The thyroid can only, by this means, reach its normal level of functioning and remain at that point. The increase in the circulation of blood to the upper parts of the body in this posture is strong enough to bring about the marvelous improvements that we speak of, but it can never become extreme.

It is always difficult for the heart to pump the blood through the parts of the body above it in a manner that provides correct and sufficiently strong circulation in those areas. As a consequence, the organs and glands of the face and head are invariably lacking in proper circulation. This is largely responsible for wrinkling and sagging conditions of the skin of the face and for the loss of hair in men.

Only the tendency to become bald if certain conditions are present is inherited by men. The actual loss of hair depends upon the conditions that arise and whether one or more of those conditions are strong enough to make this tendency physically manifest itself. The main condition that generally exists which can affect men with an inherited tendency to baldness is lack of proper blood circulation in the scalp.

The SHOULDER STAND increases in a mild and controlled manner the circulation of blood through the entire head. This improves the complexion and overall condition of the skin of the face, improves the health of the salivary glands, tends to improve the functioning of the eyes and ears, and actually stimulates and refreshes the brain. Your blood is the carrier of physical nourishment, and your brain, especially after a long day of physical and mental activity, is generally starved for nourishment. The SHOULDER STAND overcomes mental fatigue by allowing the blood to drain through the network of capillaries and blood vessels that run through the brain.

This improved circulation through the brain, as well as through the whole organism, is health-giving to the highest degree to the entire nervous system.

The Yogis also maintain that hardening of the arteries of the brain can be prevented through the years by the practice of the SHOULDER STAND.

THE HEAD STAND

· Refreshes the brain
· Helps prevent baldness
· Improves general circulation

The HEAD STAND is identified with Yoga more than nearly any other technique. It is little understood and has been often ridiculed good-naturedly by those who do not know of its effects upon the body and mind. Here you will learn the practical health-giving value of this venerable technique.

If you adhere to the following instructions and the practice schedule, you will find that the HEAD STAND is easy to master.

Use a folded towel or other padding to place your head upon while performing this posture.

1. Kneel down with your knees and heels together and place

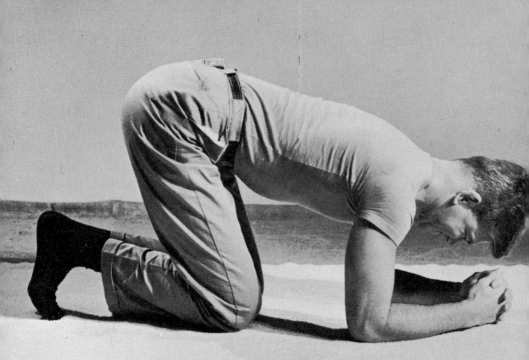

Figure 58

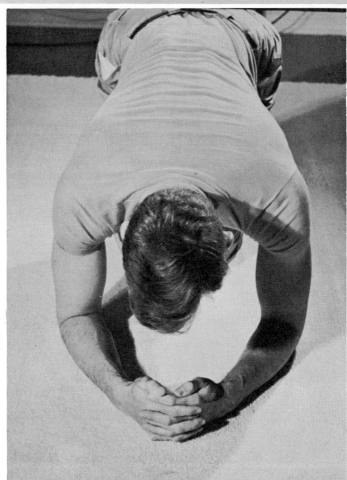

Figure 59

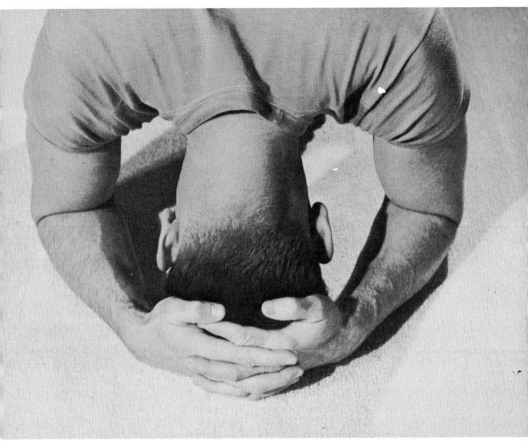

Figure 60

your arms on the floor before you in the triangular position shown in Figures 58 and 59.

2. Place your head with the top on the mat so that the back or base of your skull fits against your intertwined fingers. (Figure 60.)

3. Lifting your knees off the floor, walk slowly forward on tiptoe until your knees are touching your chest or as close to touching your chest as you can bring them. (Figures 61 and 62.)

4. Now push gently and delicately up and forward with your toes until the weight of your body shifts from your toes and head

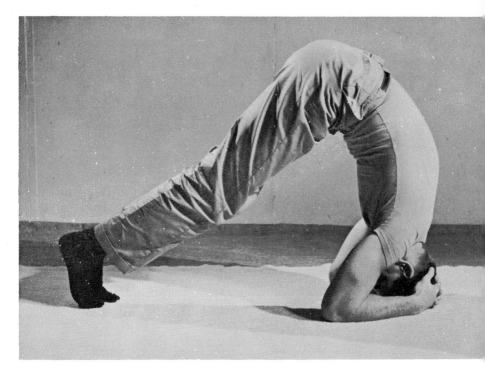

Figure 61

Figure 62

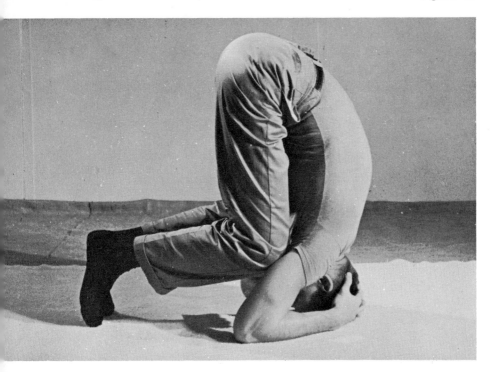

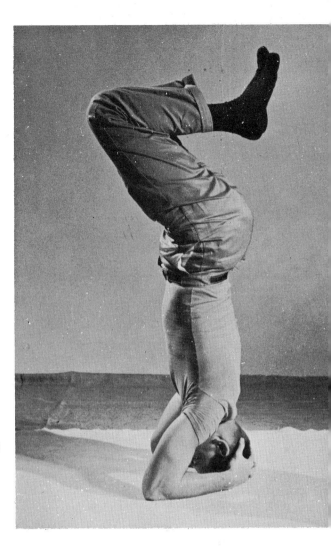

Figure 63

to your head and arms alone. Your feet will leave the floor and you will be in the position shown in Figure 63.

5. You are now in a partial or modified HEAD STAND. This is the position in which you will practice the HEAD STAND at first. Hold this position for ten seconds. Add ten seconds a week until you are holding this inverted posture for sixty seconds. Do this once a day.

6. When you have held this partial or modified HEAD STAND posture for sixty seconds, then begin to practice straightening your legs up.

If you will note the triangular base for the HEAD STAND formed by the arms and head on the floor, it becomes apparent that you have actually more balanced support in this posture than when you stand upright on your feet with your heels together.

It is essential that you straighten your legs with the utmost slowness. Only in this way can you truly master this technique. While counting to yourself, straighten your legs an inch at a time. Lift them an inch, make certain of your balance, then lift them another inch, and so on. If you proceed swiftly from the modified position of the HEAD STAND to the complete posture as depicted in Figures 64 and 65, you will never gain the true and perfect mastery of balance and control.

Coming out of the HEAD STAND correctly is as important as going into it correctly. Once again, as throughout all of Yoga, *slow motion* is the key.

7. Fold your legs, first at the knees and then at the hips, until your knees are once again close to or against your chest as in Figure 62.

You must make certain that your feet touch the floor very gently. Only this will assure your attaining the control of your body which is essential in the HEAD STAND. In coming out of the HEAD STAND, your feet must never strike the floor with a thud. Work toward this control. If you practice your partial or modified position with the correct slowness and gentleness, it should be simple for you to continue having this control when coming out of the complete HEAD STAND.

It is impossible for you to injure yourself in the HEAD STAND if you follow the instructions correctly.

After you come out of the HEAD STAND, it is important that you remain in a resting position for at least one minute. If you rest longer, it is even better for you. The pressure of your blood flow has been altered sufficiently during your time in the HEAD STAND to make it harmful for you to sit or stand up immediately upon coming down. Give your circulation time to readjust itself. This corresponds with the wise principle of resting for a short interval after performing any Yoga technique.

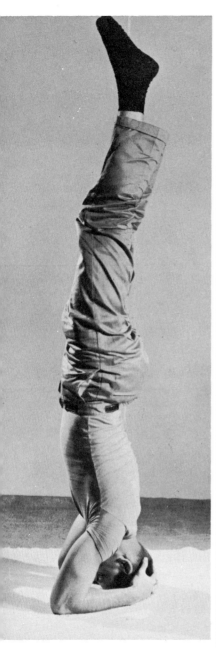

Figure 64

Figure 65

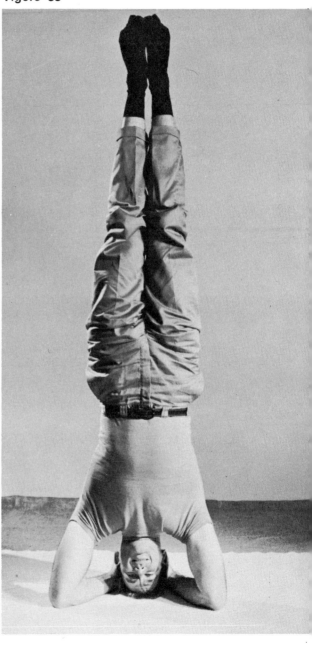

Practice Schedule

Do the HEAD STAND once a day in the afternoon. When you are able to hold the complete HEAD STAND as in Figure 65 for three minutes, you may perform the HEAD STAND in the morning if you happen to prefer that time. In the beginning, however, let the HEAD STAND work for you in counteracting the effect of the day-long pull of gravity upon your body.

Remember, build the partial HEAD STAND (Figure 63) up to sixty seconds. Then practice straightening your legs up according to instruction.

Continue adding ten seconds a week until you are holding this posture for three minutes. If you particularly enjoy this technique at that point, you may feel free to add twenty seconds a week to the time duration from then on and build up to five minutes.

Benefits

The therapeutic benefits of the HEAD STAND are the same as those of the SHOULDER STAND, only varying in degree of intensity.

Its effect upon the thyroid gland is milder than that of the SHOULDER STAND, but its effect on nearly every other part of your organism is stronger.

The wonderful results of the HEAD STAND come about mainly through its improvement of the circulation of the blood. The entire nervous system is benefited by the generally improved circulation, especially in the region of the brain.

The brain itself is vitalized and stimulated through the increased blood circulation. The heart always has a difficult time pumping blood to the head and face, and these are nearly always deficient in circulation. Persons have testified to the effect that their mental faculties—memory, alertness, sharpness of perception, etc.—have improved with continued practice of the HEAD STAND.

The pineal and pituitary glands in the brain are nourished by the stimulated circulation of blood through the blood vessels and capillaries of the brain.

The increase of blood flow through the head affects the eyes and ears very much and has been known to help overcome pathological conditions in these vital and precious organs.

The HEAD STAND definitely helps prevent baldness and stops falling hair by improving the circulation in the scalp. To the Yogi, only the tendency to become bald is inherited; actually becoming bald depends upon certain conditions. The main condition that induces baldness in a person with this tendency or predisposition is improper blood supply in the scalp. By employing the HEAD STAND you ensure the nourishment of the roots of the hair and consequently their vitality and health. Gray hair has even been known to change back to its original dark color because of the practice of this posture.

THE ABDOMINAL CONTRACTION

- Eliminates constipation
  - Reduces excessive weight in the abdomen
    - Massages and stimulates all visceral organs

The ABDOMINAL CONTRACTION is one of the most invaluable techniques known to man for the promotion and maintenance of the health of internal organs. Nearly every gland and organ of

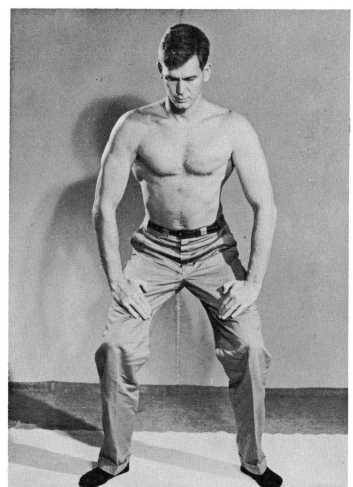

Figure 66

87

the entire visceral region is reached and benefited by this technique. Its direct effects upon the colon are incredibly therapeutic. It has been used for thousands of years by people who have existed in every conceivable condition and way of life, and has always given the same positive results.

This technique can be performed standing, squatting or sitting.

1. Stand with your feet approximately shoulder width apart. Bend your legs slightly at the knees. Place the palms of your

Figure 67

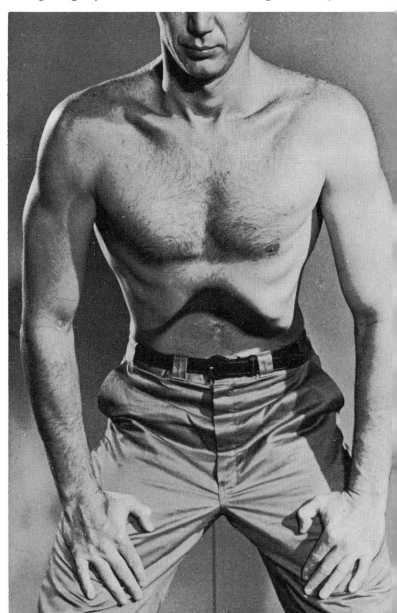

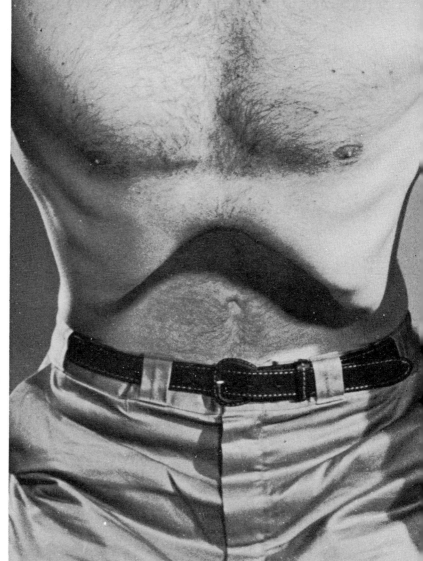

hands upon the upper part of your thighs with your fingers point-ing inward. Now support as much of the weight of your body as you can with your arms, leaning, as it were, upon your braced arms. In this position the abdominal muscles should feel a relaxed sensation. This is the stance. (Figure 66.)

2. When you are in this stance, expel all the air out of your lungs through your mouth with a loud whistling sound. When all the air has been thus blown out of your lungs, hold the air out by

not allowing any inhalation to take place throughout the performing of the abdominal movements.

3. With the stance correct and the air held *out* of your lungs, now *pull in and up* with the abdomen. This should take but an instant. Pull the abdominal region in and up as far as you can and then push it somewhat vigorously out again. Once you get the feel of the correct stance and of holding the breath out, you should notice in your own body the same great hollow indentation of the abdomen as in Figures 67, 67A and 67B. When the air is

Figure 67B

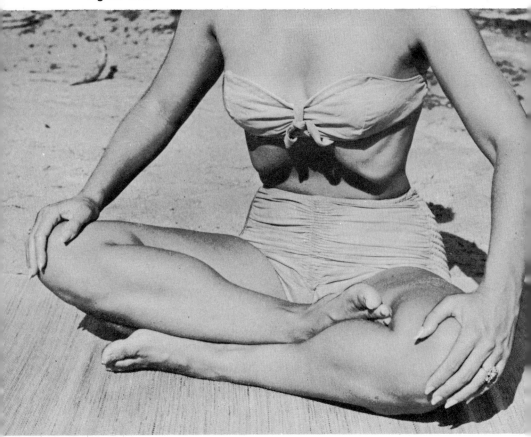

blown out of the lungs in the manner instructed, a vacuum is formed in the visceral region by the bottom of the lungs. The abdominal wall is drawn up into this vacuum, creating the hollow space observable from the outside.

The technique so far has been as follows:

a) Assume the correct stance.

b) Blow all the air out of the lungs.

c) Pull the abdomen in and up vigorously and release it the same way.

This should be repeated five times before taking a breath. In other words, once you execute the lifting of the abdomen in and up (which process should take about one second), you should repeat the movement in-out, in-out, in-out, in-out. Then stand erectly and inhale fully to resume your normal breathing.

This will be called *one set of five contractions.*

Practice Schedule

The doing of five contractions in one breath retention and then the inhalation and catching of your breath will be repeated five times. Your schedule of practicing the ABDOMINAL CONTRACTION will commence with five sets of five contractions and continue as follows:

Second day: Six sets of five contractions.
Third day: Seven sets of five contractions. Continue in like man-
ner until you are doing
Sixth day: Ten sets of five contractions.
From this point on you will progress as follows:
Seventh day: Ten sets of six contractions.
Eighth day: Ten sets of seven contractions. Continue in like
manner until you are doing
Eleventh day: Ten sets of ten contractions.

Note the gradual increase. This gradual increase in the appli-cation of the technique is practiced throughout the science of Yoga and in as methodical a fashion as possible. The more methodically and mechanically you practice Yoga, the more quickly and efficiently you will obtain the desired results. Indeed, haphazard practice brings little if any results.

By the time you have thus gradually increased the number of ABDOMINAL CONTRACTIONS to ten sets of ten lifts, your abdominal muscles have been toned and are prepared to perform that amount. Also, your body has had the necessary time and practice to adjust itself to the keeping of the breath out of the lungs and can easily accommodate your doing ten contractions in a single breath.

You will then be doing one hundred abdominal lifts, having built up to it gradually. This should take you not much more than three minutes to perform.

Benefits

The ABDOMINAL CONTRACTION is a hygienic technique. It is recommended to practice it in the morning before breakfast. It can be practiced or repeated with equal physical benefit at any other time of the day, provided that the stomach is empty. The ABDOMINAL CONTRACTION *must be practiced on an empty stomach*. Before meals is the best time. Otherwise wait at least ninety minutes after eating before practicing it. Even then, if you feel full, wait until that feeling is gone.

If you have a cardiac condition, or any other serious negative internal condition, consult your physician before attempting this technique.

Here is a Yoga technique, the profundity of which makes it deserving of an entire treatise in itself. Much medical research has been done on this technique in India as well as in the Western world, and all the therapeutic claims made for it throughout the ages have been scientifically verified.

We Americans eat a devitalized diet: altered foods, the life of which has been destroyed. As a consequence, as always, of improper eating plus lack of natural body use, the functioning of various parts of our organism has become impaired. One such vital part is the colon, or large intestine.

There is a wavelike motion which moves through the entire alimentary canal—that continuous tube which extends from the mouth to the anus—and whose function is to pass nutriment along the tube. This movement is known as peristaltic action. Due to the reasons given above, the peristaltic action of the colon has, in an enormous percentage of people, become sluggish. They can no longer eliminate waste matter properly. They suffer from many and often terrible illnesses because of this condition, and they are forced to spend millions of dollars each year on patent laxatives. This is the malady of constipation.

All that a laxative can do is temporarily relieve constipation. It can never cure it. Indeed, laxatives are in most instances addicting and serve only to make the colon weaker and weaker and make the poor sufferer more dependent every day on these chemicals. Once again, outside aids can at best only temporarily alleviate negative bodily conditions.

Correct alteration of the diet has a much better effect upon a large intestine that no longer functions properly. But this varies in effect and takes considerable time and effort to arrive at.

There is only one cure for a negative condition, and that is removal of the cause of it. The immediate cause of constipation here is the malfunctioning of the peristaltic action of the colon.

The ABDOMINAL CONTRACTION corrects the sluggish peristaltic action of the colon and brings it back to normal so that it does its work of eliminating toxic waste matter properly. Here again Yoga accomplishes its physical result by means of stretching. The ABDOMINAL CONTRACTION actually manipulates and stretches the colon in a rhythmical and perfectly natural fashion and, in so doing, stimulates it, strengthens it, and restores its normal peristaltic action.

The Yogi will state that you need never suffer from common constipation again if you practice the ABDOMINAL CONTRACTION as instructed.

To add to the strength of this technique, you may drink a glassful of water with the juice of half a lemon in it before performing it. Only do this if you feel that it is necessary.

At the same time, the ABDOMINAL CONTRACTION massages and stimulates the small intestine, liver, spleen, pancreas, gall bladder, stomach, and the reproductive glands and organs.

It strengthens the abdominal wall, reducing weight in that area, and helps raise the misplaced or even prolapsed visceral organs back into their normal place which is high in the viscera and braced by a firm wall of muscle.

It aids in reducing weight in the waist and hips.

This technique will be worth many times more than the price you paid for it. Practice it daily and help ensure the health and well-being of your internal organs. Remember, health is internal and is not synonymous with large muscles or physical prowess.

NETI

· Cleanses the nasal passages
· Increases resistance to colds
· Clears and alerts the mind in the morning

This age-old technique should prove to be a blessing to every sufferer from chronic negative condition of the nasal passages.

1. Fill a glass with warm water. Dissolve a pinch of salt in it.

2. To perform NETI on the left nostril, pour this salt water into your cupped left hand, holding your hand as in Figure 68.

3. Bring your left hand up to your face so that the ring and middle fingers can press against the right nostril and shut it while you dip the left nostril into the water. (Figure 68.)

4. Inhale *very gently* through the left nostril, which is in the water.

5. Now tilt your head very slowly back, holding the suction against the water, until a few drops of the water roll through the nostril and into the mouth.

Spit this water out.

The gentle suction and the slow tilting of the head back is the key to this technique. If you apply anything but the most extreme gentleness, the water will be sucked up into the top of the nasal passage, striking the tender nerves there and causing a stinging sensation.

It is this unpleasant sensation which you avoid by the correct gentle practice of NETI. The manner in which you will draw the warm water through your nose as instructed here will cause the

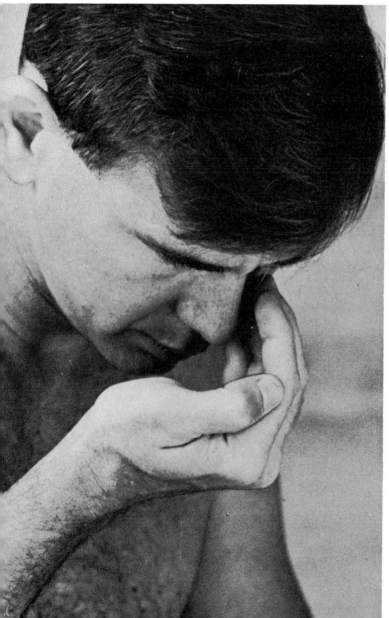

Figure 68

water to roll along the bottom and sides of the nostril and not strike that tender spot.

6. Pour the warm salt water into your cupped right hand and do the same thing to your right nostril.

Alternate this way until you have performed NETI three times on each nostril.

It is necessary for only a few drops to go through the nostrils to be expectorated in order for the results to take place.

Practice Schedule

NETI is a hygienic—cleansing—technique. It should be practiced once a day, in the morning before breakfast, preferably as part of your morning ablutions.

You may do it more than once a day *when needed* if you happen to catch a cold or have a congested nasal condition. You will find it extremely useful in helping to alleviate such conditions.

Benefits

NETI is a most ancient technique.

It cleanses the nasal passages.

When performed in the morning, it serves as a great refresher and wakes one up marvelously, promoting alertness and clarity of mind.

It toughens the membranes of the nasal passages and definitely develops resistance to colds.

It can and should be used to relieve the discomforts of colds, sinus and other conditions affecting the nasal region.

THE CLEANSING BREATH

- Cleans the lungs of impurities
  - Builds resistance to colds
    - Helps overcome the cigarette habit

Bearing in mind the fundamental rule of correct breathing, namely, that when the breath is inhaled, the abdomen expands outward and when the breath is exhaled, the abdomen contracts inward, you will learn here a breathing technique which demonstrates a quick, forceful example of this basic bodily movement.

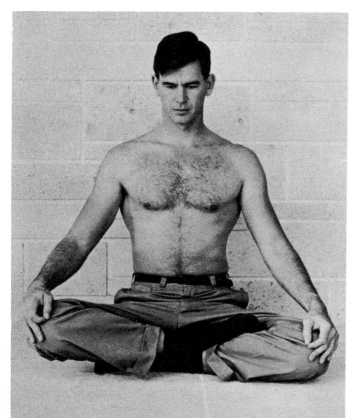

Figure 69

97

1. Sit in the crosslegged posture which is most comfortable for you. Breathe normally.

2. Expanding your abdomen only (making a big "belly" in order to bring the diaphragm down and forward), inhale about a third of a lungful of air. (Figure 69.)

This is the preparatory condition for beginning a round of CLEANSING BREATHS.

3. *Forcefully* pull in your abdomen and at the same time *forcefully* and quickly expel all the air in your lungs through your nose. (Figure 70.)

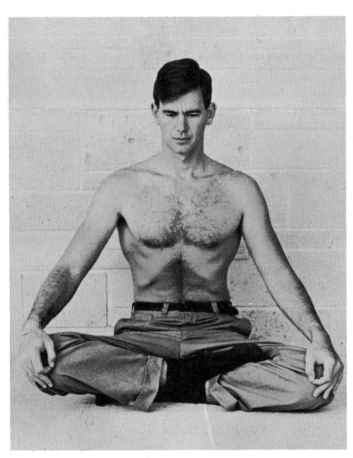

Figure 70

4. Immediately take another partial breath through your nose while extending your abdomen outward once again. (Figure 69.)

5. When the abdomen cannot protrude any further, quickly and forcefully expel the air out through your nose and with the same quick forcefulness pull your abdomen in.

You will be practicing this technique in a series of a certain number of inhalations and exhalations. A steady rhythm will invariably be established. The accent should be upon the forceful *expulsion* of air through the nose and the corresponding vigorous pulling in of the abdominal muscles. The inhalation and expansion of the abdominal muscles is a more relaxed movement.

Practice Schedule

Each CLEANSING BREATH—one exhalation and one inhalation—should take from one to two seconds.

Do ten such CLEANSING BREATHS one after the other as one round of CLEANSING BREATHS. Follow each round of CLEANSING BREATHS with one COMPLETE BREATH. (See p. 100.)

Do two rounds of CLEANSING BREATHS for the first week.

Add one more round of ten CLEANSING BREATHS each week until you are doing six rounds of ten CLEANSING BREATHS, each round followed by a COMPLETE BREATH.

The CLEANSING BREATH is extremely hygienic and is best done in the morning before breakfast.

It is also well to do it *preceding* your regular daily Yoga workout.

Benefits

Those who smoke will find this technique especially useful. Many persons have asked me, "Can I study Yoga and hope to gain its ultimate results? I have the smoking habit and cannot break it." My answer has always been, "You do not have to stop smoking before you can seriously practice the physical aspect of Yoga. In fact, if you practice Yoga, with special emphasis on the CLEANSING BREATH, for a sufficient length of time—usually at least six months—you will find that one day upon picking up a cigarette you will be unable to smoke it. The lungs will have been cleansed of coal tar residues and other impurities to such an extent that the organism will be revolted by the cigarette fumes and never crave them again." Such is the power of the CLEANSING BREATH. And when this occurs, you are gaining health and losing only a bad habit. Thus these simple, ancient, natural techniques have the power to accomplish what the strongest efforts of will power as well as many forms of therapy cannot accomplish.

Those who do not have the smoking habit are still subjected to an age of gasoline and noxious chemical fumes. The CLEANSING BREATH and other Yogic breathing techniques have the ability to counteract the toxic, nerve-harming and vitality-draining effects of these impurities.

The CLEANSING BREATH literally "rubs" phlegm, coal tar residues and impurities loose from the respiratory system and enables them to be expelled.

Steady, regular practice of the CLEANSING BREATH can relieve minor respiratory ailments such as colds and coughs. It aids in the draining of congested sinuses.

The CLEANSING BREATH, when practiced in conjunction with the COMPLETE BREATH, has a delightful awakening effect in the morning. It refreshes the system.

The diaphragm is developed and the abdominal wall is strengthened and made taut and tough.

THE COMPLETE BREATH

· Purifies the blood
· Increases vitality
· Develops the chest

1. Sit crosslegged on your mat—SIMPLE POSTURE, HALF LOTUS or FULL LOTUS. Rest your wrists on your knees. Sit erectly, your nose on a line with your navel and your ears on a line with your shoulders.

All breathing is done through the nose in Yoga unless specifically instructed otherwise in certain techniques.

It is necessary to master three bodily movements in order to be able to perform the COMPLETE BREATH. These three movements are explained in steps 2, 3 and 4.

2. Exhale slightly through your nose. Now commence inhaling through your nose while making the following movement:

Push down and out with your diaphragm.

The diaphragm is the sheet of muscle that separates your chest cavity from your abdomen. The process of pushing this diaphragm

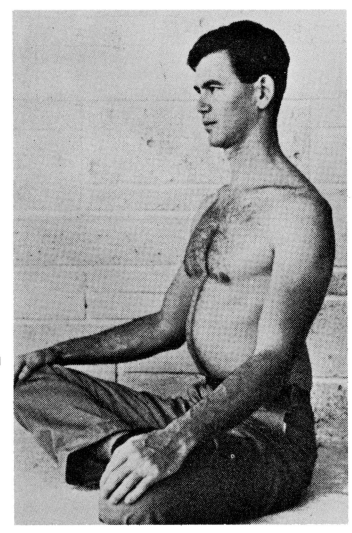

Figure 71

down and out consists of the simple technique of "making a big belly." Push your abdominal region out as far as you can. This automatically draws the diaphragm outward. Remember to push your abdomen downward at the same time. Do not be disappointed or in doubt if you see no noticeable protrusion of your abdomen upon first trying this movement. The muscles involved will regain their natural resiliency in time.

To begin your formal practice of the COMPLETE BREATH, count five seconds to make this first movement. (Figure 71.)

3. Still inhaling slowly, smoothly and quietly, in the next five seconds perform the following movement:

Bring your extended abdomen *in* until it feels taut and at the

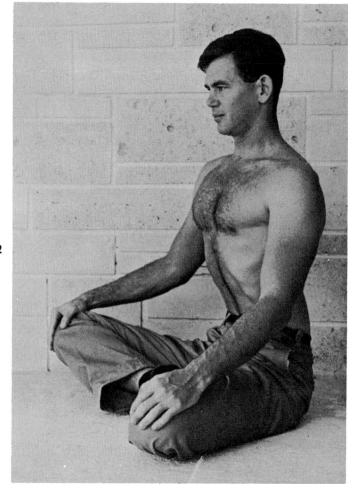

Figure 72

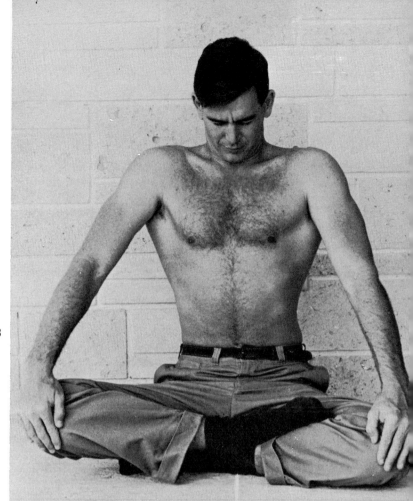

Figure 73

same time spread your ribs, expanding your entire rib cage. (Figure 72.)

To expand your rib cage correctly, push forward with your breastbone and attempt to spread your ribs outward at the sides. As with most of these techniques, you will get the "feel" of it very quickly and you will then know how correctly you are performing it.

4. The third bodily movement of the COMPLETE BREATH is as follows:

Still inhaling slowly and quietly, place the fingertips of each hand upon the corresponding knee, raise your elbows as high into the air as they can go without removing your fingertips from contact with your knees, and then lift your shoulders up as far as you can, as if you would have your neck disappear between them. (Figure 73.)

The abdomen is pulled tightly in at this point and held tightly in until the next breath begins, when the diaphragm must once again be extended down and out.

This third movement, ending with the complete raising of the shoulders, will also be performed to the count of five seconds.

So far, one slow, quiet inhalation of breath has been taken for the count of fifteen seconds. During this fifteen-second inhalation, the three movements just described have been performed, each of the movements taking five seconds. Both the movements and the inhalations are to be executed in a *smooth, continuous manner.*

5. At this point you will hold your breath in for the count of ten seconds.

Note: Three special techniques are to be performed with the body *while* the breath is being *retained.* These are:

The Chin Lock. This movement consists of lowering your chin as soon as the COMPLETE BREATH has been inhaled and has begun to be retained until your chin rests firmly against the notch formed by the insides of your collarbones and the top of your breastbone (known as the jugular notch). The chin is held against this jugular notch until the breath has been retained for the prescribed count. (Figure 74.)

The Abdominal Lock. This movement is already being performed during breath retention. It consists of pulling in and up with the abdomen and holding the abdominal wall tightly in and high as previously instructed.

The Anal Lock. This manipulation consists of closing the anal sphincters tightly by squeezing the buttocks together and drawing the anal sphincters upward.

6. The breath is now expelled in a controlled manner, *slowly,* smoothly and *quietly,* the shoulders being lowered at the same rate in which they were raised. The exhalation should be per-

formed in this quiet, controlled manner to the count of fifteen seconds. The Chin Lock is released, and the head is raised until you are looking forward as in the beginning.

Summary of COMPLETE BREATH technique:

Inhale to the count of fifteen, performing the three movements as described.

Retain your breath for the count of ten, practicing the three locks as instructed.

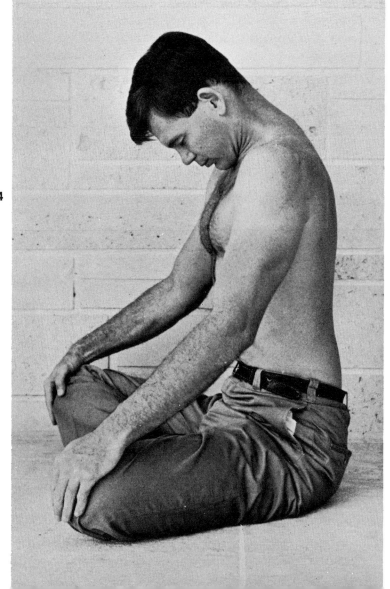

Figure 74

Exhale to the count of fifteen with no special movements, simply relaxing the posture that was assumed. Do not, however, "collapse" out of the posture or allow your breath to gush out. Control the coming out of any Yoga technique. This is essential to success in Yoga. When you have finished exhaling and are ready to inhale the next COMPLETE BREATH, you should be in the same erect and correct sitting position as when you began.

Your body will quickly adapt itself to these new postures and movements which you are teaching it.

Practice Schedule

Do the COMPLETE BREATH three to five times after your regular Yoga practice period but before you perform the ALTERNATE NOSTRIL BREATHING and before you practice any of your Mental (Raja Yoga) techniques.

The COMPLETE BREATH may and should be performed as many times as you are able during the day. Simply do not practice the exaggerated movement of raising your shoulders, as you would in the privacy of your home.

You may practice it while sitting, standing, walking or even driving your car. No one need know you are breathing in this complete manner, due to the elimination of the shoulder raising and the formal breath retention with the locks. The COMPLETE BREATH is the correct and natural way of breathing. By practicing it both formally at home and informally when in public, you will reap incalculable benefits to your health and state of mind.

The principle behind the physical movements of the COMPLETE BREATH can be stated in one sentence: You can only be certain of filling a sack completely by opening the sack *before* pouring in the contents.

Let us use simple, practical examples to illustrate what we mean. Imagine a grocery bag which you wish to fill with grain. Then imagine that the bottom half of this paper bag is crumpled and squeezed together. If you were to pour grain, no matter how finely ground, into this bag, only a few grains would trickle through to the bottom. The bulk of the grain would start filling the bag from the point just above the crumpled area.

In this same manner, if the bottom of the lungs are contracted, air that is inhaled will not reach the bottom. The lungs will commence to fill from a point midway or higher. It is then impossible to get full use of the lungs.

The point is that *if you want to fill the lungs with air, you must first open the lungs so that the air being inhaled will go directly to the bottom of the lungs and fill up the lungs from the bottom and from the farthest recesses.*

We have seen the person at the beach who is going to take what he believes to be a complete or "deep" breath. He takes a mighty inhalation, making a tremendous chest and at the same time pulling his abdomen up and in. You can now see the fallacy of such a method. Pulling the abdomen in compresses the lower part of the lungs. Only by the movements of the COMPLETE BREATH that you have now learned can the lungs be opened in the correct fashion so as to enable the air to fill them completely from the bottom.

Extending the abdomen, which pushes the diaphragm out and down, frees the lower portion of the lungs so that they can be filled. Spreading the ribs as in the second part of the inhalation movement allows the middle portion of the lungs to be filled completely. Raising the shoulders in the third part of the inhalation enables the air to fill the upper portion of the lungs and reach those seldom-aerated lobes which are so susceptible to tuberculosis.

We are the most scientifically enlightened country in the world. Yet, from childhood on, nowhere in our educational system is correct breathing taught. The magnitude of this error is enormous, and the price we pay for the lack of this knowledge has for some years been, in terms of health, a national tragedy.

The average person breathes far too quickly—from fifteen to twenty-two times a minute—and far too shallowly—the air trickling in usually no further than the top third of the lung. No wonder the body is devitalized when it is kept continuously famished for its primary source of nourishment and energy, the air. *The slower and more completely you breathe, the longer you will live and the healthier you will be.* Look to nature. The animals—like the elephant, the turtle and the parrot—who have the longest life spans are the ones who breathe the slowest. Those creatures who breathe the most rapidly—the mouse, the hare—are characterized by short life spans.

Also observe how the slow-breathing animals are the calmest while the fast-breathing animals are the most nervous. We will go more deeply into this aspect of breathing when we cover in detail the subject of the relation of the breath to the mind and to the nervous system.

Thus breathing *completely*, as the Yogis have for thousands of years, will:

1. Re-educate your body to breathe in the natural slow and complete manner, and

2. Produce profoundly healthful effects upon your organism.

The COMPLETE BREATH is man's *natural* way of breathing. Note certain primitive people who live a life very close to nature. You have observed how peculiarly enlarged their abdomens are, even though the individual might be a towering example of physical leanness and strength. This is not a malformity. This is the powerful muscular development of the abdominal and diaphragmatic region due to a lifetime of correct natural breathing. Note as well how infants and little children breathe. Observe them when they are asleep and you will see the abdominal region move in and out as they breathe, not the upper chest. They breathe in the natural manner of man, not in the sickly shallow gasps with which nearly everyone around us breathes.

The correct Yogic complete inhalation will fill your lungs to capacity. Thus will you receive many times the usual amount of oxygen and precious Life-Force.

Correctly retaining the air in your lungs for a number of seconds ensures that the greatest possible quantity of oxygen enters your bloodstream. It also gives your body a greater chance to expel waste matter carried by the blood into the hollow cavity of the lungs.

Correct exhalation ensures that all the waste matter is expelled. (Keeping your abdominal wall drawn tightly in throughout the exhalation contracts the lower portion of your lungs so that the last of the stale impurities are squeezed from your lung sacs.) The complete exhalation also enables the next inhalation to take place in a truly complete manner.

Benefits

The COMPLETE BREATH purifies the blood and improves its quality through complete oxygenation.

By strengthening the lung tissue itself this technique increases resistance to colds and other respiratory ailments.

The controlled, rhythmical and complete movements involved tend in time to enable the practitioner of Yoga to relieve colds and the discomforts of other negative respiratory conditions by means of the application of the COMPLETE BREATH.

Your nervous system is strengthened by regular practice of this technique because of the increased amount of Life-Force, or *Prana*, which is brought into your system. The subject of *Prana* will be dealt with in more detail in a future chapter.

The chest cavity and the diaphragm are developed and strengthened.

The COMPLETE BREATH increases vitality and endurance, improves the complexion and makes the mind clear and alert.

ALTERNATE NOSTRIL BREATHING

· Quiets the body and mind
· Calms and strengthens the nerves
· Imparts emotional control

Here is the essence of Hatha Yoga.

1. Sit in your most comfortable crosslegged posture.

2. Hold your right hand as depicted in Figure 75.

3. Place your right thumb lightly against your right nostril, *not* closing the nostril. Place the ring finger of that hand lightly against the left nostril, not closing it. This is the basic position and the one from which you will start.

Figure 75

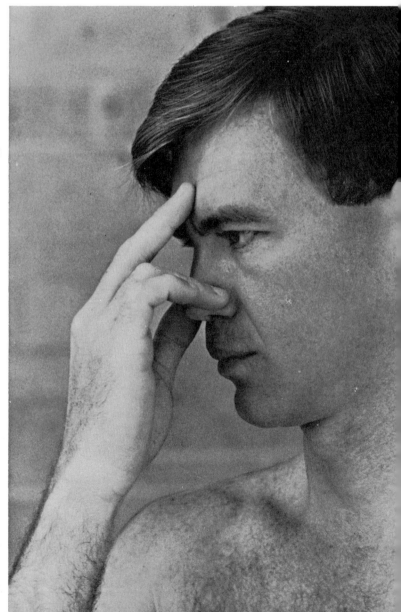

All breathing in Yoga is performed with the abdominal and chest movements of the COMPLETE BREATH. Adhere to the basic rule of natural breathing: *When the breath comes in, the stomach goes out; when the breath goes out, the stomach comes in.*

4. Exhale slightly.

5. Close your right nostril by pressing your right thumb against

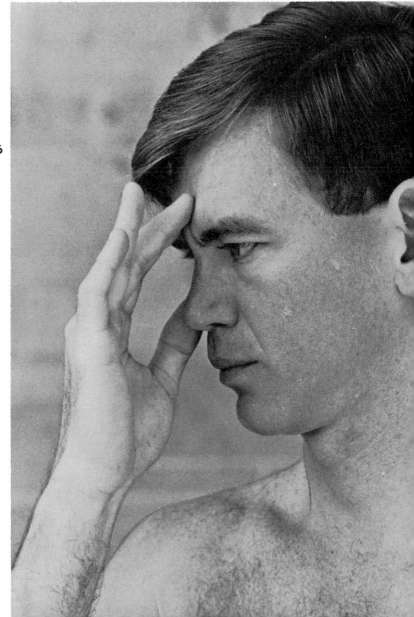

Figure 76

it. Inhale completely through your left nostril for the count of eight. (Figure 76.)

6. Close both nostrils. Retain the air inside your body for the count of eight.

Once this technique, through practice, has become automatic with you and you do not have to think about the basic movements of the fingers, you should apply the three locks to it that you

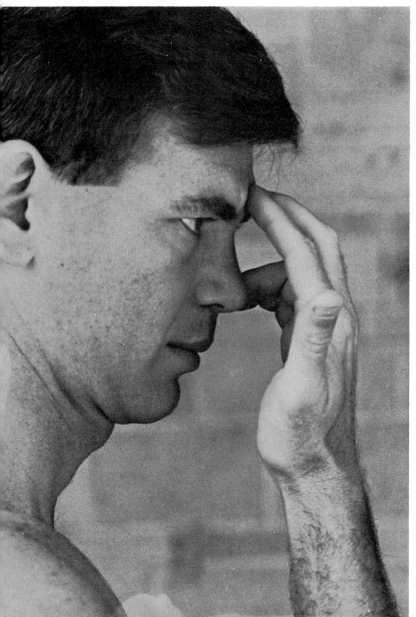

Figure 77

learned in the Complete Breath. The Chin Lock, especially, should be applied in all breath retention.

7. Open your right nostril by raising your right thumb off it. Exhale through your right nostril for the count of eight. (Figure 77.)

8. Without pause, inhale through your right nostril for the count of eight.

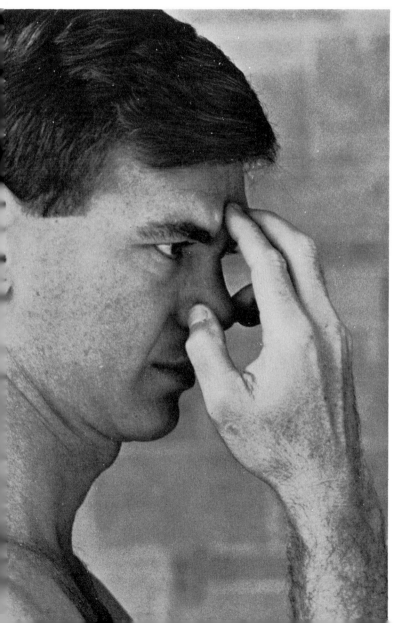

Figure 78

9. Close both nostrils and retain the breath for the count of eight. (Figure 78.)

10. Open your left nostril by raising your ring finger off it. Exhale through your left nostril for the count of eight.

This is one round of ALTERNATE NOSTRIL BREATHING.

Practice Schedule

The ALTERNATE NOSTRIL BREATHING is most beneficial when performed shortly before retiring at night. When practiced as part of your regular Yoga workout period, it should always be the last technique.

Practice the ALTERNATE NOSTRIL BREATHING technique to the count of eight-eight-eight as instructed here.

Do seven rounds each time you practice it.

Benefits

The ALTERNATE BREATHING technique calms both body and mind. This is not the type of so-called tranquilization that comes with sleep, narcosis or hypnosis. This is an alert calm, based on emotional balance as well as a delightful relaxing sensation imparted to the nervous system itself.

The ALTERNATE NOSTRIL BREATHING should always be resorted to in times of emotional upset or anticipated emotional stress. When bad news or a negative situation arises and your emotional body dominates your nature, you should get away by yourself at once and do from five to seven rounds of ALTERNATE NOSTRIL BREATHING. You will be gratified by the results. Your emotional balance will be restored. If you face a situation where you will need full emotional and nervous self-control—appearing in public, undergoing tests, etc.—you should do the same. ALTERNATE BREATHING is the supreme counter-agent to fear, anger, anxiety and other such states.

This technique balances powerful yet subtle forces which work in and through the body and in so doing strengthens the entire nervous system. Nervous disorders have been alleviated by use of this technique.

It has been used with much success in normalizing high and low blood pressure conditions.

Numerous cases of insomnia have been completely alleviated by the correct use of ALTERNATE NOSTRIL BREATHING.

PART TWO
FOOD AND NUTRITION

THE VIEWPOINT OF YOGA
ON FOOD AND NUTRITION

The use of food by human beings goes far beyond the principle of eat or die. It has to do with the quality of living. By eating incorrectly you can deteriorate your body, decrease your vitality, make your body susceptible to and actually create major diseases. These conditions bring corresponding states of mind—depression, fatigue, anxiety. The individual in such a state loses his or her ability to develop the potential greatness or gifts within him.

By eating correctly, negative conditions are removed and prevented, resulting in vitality, energy, lightness, optimism and the positive effects of such traits upon the world you live in.

What is correct eating? What is incorrect eating?

At the present time in this country and many other countries there exist a number of schools of thought about nutrition. The two main camps of contention are those who believe in what we can call the natural food principle and those who do not. There are differences of theory and opinion in each of these camps.

It is the Yogi's opinion that the population of the United States at present is suffering terrible effects from wrong eating habits. The following five categories will account for nearly all the negative conditions and misfortunes, individual and national, that our eating habits have brought upon us.

1. *Overeating.* We eat too much. Instead of putting the right amount of really nourishing food into our bodies, we stuff ourselves with nearly indigestible material and even more indigestible mixtures.

119

Just because a mechanism needs oil it does not follow that the more oil you put into it the better. On the contrary, put too much oil in a machine and you can damage or destroy it. Your body is a precision instrument, finer and more exact than any that could ever be created by man. Think of the damage that is being done to it by overloading it three times a day whether it needs it or not.

2. *Devitalized foods.* The foods we do eat are deficient in nutritional value. Fruits and vegetables are grown with inorganic (usually chemically manufactured) fertilizer. The consequence of the use of this type of fertilizer is that food thus grown is lacking in the proper quantity and *quality* of minerals and nutritional elements.

Pasteurization and similar processes devitalize the foods to which they are applied—milk, cheeses and dried fruits of various kinds.

Canning and freezing decrease and often nearly destroy the life-giving qualities of foods.

When foods are devitalized, the solution is not simply to eat more of them to make up for the devitalization. The quality itself is damaged and cannot be made up by quantity.

3. *Poison sprays.* Our weapons against insects and pests that eat our fruit and vegetable crops are more harmful to us in the long run than the destruction wrought by the insects themselves. Poison sprays are not easily washed off by any means. Besides this, a great quantity of the poisons fall upon the ground. These deadly and often cancer-producing poisons soak into the ground, are absorbed with moisture by the plants and tree roots and eventually find their way into the inside of the fruit or vegetable itself.

The poison and insecticide manufacturers state that this quantity is too small to harm us, but the truth is that the effects are cumulative through the years and strike us with frightful effect in time.

4. *Eating improper combinations of foods.* Applying the principle that "it all goes into the same place" is responsible for an

enormous percentage of indigestion, constipation, ulcer and acidity cases and many other serious maladies. It may all go into the same place, but it certainly does different things there, according to the mixture or combination of foods.

It is essential to know which foods can be eaten together in order to get the most health and vitality out of them and to avoid negative conditions brought about by putting into your stomach foods that simply do not belong there together.

Proper and improper combinations of foods will be explained in some detail shortly.

5. *Ignorance of the correct principles of eating and nutrition.* Explanation and examples of the correct principles of eating and nutrition form the bulk of the remainder of this exposition.

There is a subtle force which pervades all of the universe and everything that exists in the universe. The name given to this force in Sanskrit is *Prana*. We shall translate the word *Prana* as "Life-Force."

Everything is permeated with the Life-Force. Animated, or what we call "living" or "organic" matter, is kept in the living state by the Life-Force that functions in and through it. If the Life-Force functions in an organism, it breathes, moves and is alive. If the Life-Force leaves an organism, that organism ceases to breathe and move and is dead. This immeasurable, mysterious, primal force is the sustainer of life. And it is to obtain this force and to keep this force functioning in us that we breathe, drink, eat, sleep and use the light of the sun. The purpose of taking nourishment in any and all of these five forms is to keep the Life-Force entering and moving in us.

The more Life-Force we have functioning through us, the more alive we are in every conceivable way. Improper eating diminishes the Life-Force in us. Correct eating increases our Life-Force.

Since before written history, the Yogis have adhered to a wonderful concept regarding the effects of food upon the physical, mental and spiritual condition of man. This is the concept of the *gunas*.

The Sanskrit word *guna* is generally translated as "a primary quality." The notion is as follows.

There are three primary qualities from which everything that exists is built. Everything that exists has all three of these qualities in its makeup, but one will always be dominant. The first of these *gunas*, or qualities, is called *tamas*. *Tamas guna* is the tendency for things to become dense and inert. A physical example of the dominance of *tamas guna* is the element lead, the most dense and inert of substances on the scale of life.

The opposite quality, or *sattva guna*, is the tendency for things to expand, become less dense. A physical example of this is the expansion, diffusion and rising of gas.

The middle quality, or *rajas guna*, is the predisposition in all things to move in either of those directions, to have to move toward density or expansion.

It is much simpler to understand this idea when we see how it is applied to human beings. For people also are composed of and represent these three primary qualities, one of which always predominates. In human beings, *tamas guna*, the principle of denseness, takes the form of ignorance, sloth and inertness and their by-products. A small percentage of the human race is predominantly tamasic by nature. An example of such people is the chronic alcoholic, such as the so-called "wino," who exists as a social phenomenon in nearly every community. Rajasic people are dominated by the principle of action motivated by the passions or emotions. This category represents the vast majority of people. Sattvic people are a small minority. They are those persons who are not dominated by their passions. Their intelligence and consciousness tend to expand. They represent the spiritual individuals of the human community.

But how does one tell if a person is dominated by the quality of *tamas* (denseness), *rajas* (passion) or *sattva* (expansion)? *It is by what he eats.*

Tamasic people tend to eat decayed or fermented foods. They prefer leftovers and foods which drain and diminish the Life-Force from an organism. Physically, their eating preferences are self-destructive. Their longevity is shortened. Their contribution to the world around them is generally negative.

Rajasic people tend to eat foods which heat the body and make the passions easily aroused. An example of this is the highly acid-forming diet of the average American and the superabundance of the meat and starch combination in our everyday diet. Irritability, temper, lusts, etc. are stimulated by rajasic foods. Their energy and physical strength, however great, is short-lived and quickly burns itself out.

Sattvic people attain the greatest peace and stability of body, mind and soul. They tend to eat foods which are light and nourishing and which cool and soothe their organisms. Fresh fruits and vegetables and other natural plant foods are preferred by them.

The profound and immensely important part of this concept is that not only do persons of these types tend toward eating foods representative of their category, but *whoever makes his diet correspond to this system will become more and more predominantly of the type his food represents.* This, of course, is not an overnight process, nor can it be accomplished in a two week "crash" program, although the first effects are definitely felt at once.

The effect of diet upon the human race has been observed by the Yogis for thousands of years. If you subsist on tamasic foods, you will develop tamasic traits of body, mind and character. The same applies to the eating of Rajasic and sattvic foods. This is because the essence as well as a considerable portion of the substance of what you eat becomes part of your organism—becomes you, so to speak, when it finally reaches the point of being absorbed into your cells.

Thus does the quality of the food you eat effect you. It alters your personality and character as easily as it determines the state of health of your body. Bearing in mind, then, that the Yogi eats to supply himself with Life-Force and to increase the sattvic (consciousness-expanding) part of his nature, we will now enter into the details of what the right human diet is.

The Natural Food Principle. It is recommended that you follow the natural food principle whenever possible. This rule, however, must be tempered with common sense. Some foods cannot be digested properly in their raw or natural state. The matter of digestion also varies from individual to individual. Just because the Yogi believes in eating foods as close as possible to their natural state, do not attempt, for example, to eat raw potatoes. Yet raw cabbage or raw corn are, when chewed sufficiently, extremely good for you and many times greater in nutritional value than when cooked.

Vegetables. Lettuce, carrots, celery, corn, cucumbers, radishes and green peppers are best eaten raw. They contain vital elements and minerals difficult to obtain in other foods. They counteract the overacidity of the body which most Americans have. Other vegetables, such as potatoes, sweet potatoes, Brussels sprouts, string beans, rhubarb and squash must be cooked. But do not, as is the unfortunate and unhealthy habit in our country, overcook them. Overcooking vegetables diminishes and often destroys their nutritional value. Vegetables should be cooked lightly so that they retain a certain amount of their natural crunchiness. A good example of properly cooked vegetables are the ones you receive in a Chinese restaurant. If a cooked vegetable is soft and limp, then you may know that it has been overcooked. The broth left from cooked vegetables is rich in vitamins and minerals and should be drunk.

Children are easily conditioned to eating vegetables raw. This is a boon to their health and also counteracts their tendency to depend on sweets for a snack. When a child wants a snack, hand him a carrot or other vegetable. They quickly develop a taste for these items.

Fruits. Fruits should always be eaten raw. You cannot overeat fruits. They cleanse the body and soothe the digestive tract. They are the richest of all foods in sugar, the most easily digested and easily absorbed form of sugar. Fruits provide energy as well as essential vitamins and nutriments.

Canning destroys nearly every good thing fruits have to offer you. Preservation in heavy syrup is just as bad. Cooked fruits are virtually dead fruits. Freezing also impairs the value of these precious foods. We classify fruits in two categories. The main distinction between them is that they are not meant to be mixed with each other and eaten at the same time.

Oranges, lemons, grapefruits, raspberries, pineapples, limes and strawberries we will call acid fruits. These are highly desirable breakfast foods because they cut through and loosen sticky mucus-like impurities which collect in the digestive tract to be expelled. The juice of acid fruits also aids the body in eliminating toxic waste matter.

Apples, bananas, grapes, melons, peaches, pears, plums and apricots we will call sweet fruits. They are highly energizing and important in promoting regularity.

Nuts. Nuts are one of the best meat substitutes. Ounce for ounce, they provide the body with more and better quality protein than meat. Never eat salted or roasted nuts. These processes render the nuts indigestible. Nuts should be chewed thoroughly—until liquefied—for the best results. Peanuts should be avoided. They are not a nut but are actually a legume like the bean. The best nuts for human consumption are walnuts, almonds, brazil nuts and cashews, raw and unprocessed.

Dried fruits. These nourishing foods are rich in minerals and are highly energizing. Avoid eating those dried fruits to which sulfur or a sulfur compound has been added as a preservative. Dried fruits mix very well with sweet fresh fruits.

As our first unit of foods under the natural food principle we have spoken about vegetables, fresh fruits, nuts and dried fruits. Nuts are only weight-producing when eaten in wrong combination, such as with meat, starches and white sugar products. When eaten in conjunction with a correct, or natural, diet they do not add weight.

The key to getting the full benefit out of food is to make sure that the food has not been tampered with by man. The more food has been tampered with by man, the more it becomes harmful and injurious. The closer to its natural state food is, the more healthful and beneficial it is for you.

The fruits, vegetables and nuts which we have just spoken about are the most sattvic of all foods available to us. That is, they cool and soothe your organism, they produce a lightness and buoyancy of body and mind. They are at the same time most healthy for you, being full of vitamins, minerals and other vital nutritional elements.

If you eliminate certain undesirable foods from your diet and replace them with these fruits and vegetables, you will note a great change both in your physical and mental states. A clarity and alertness of the mind is one of the results of changing to a more sattvic diet.

You will also find that you have access to more abundant energy. This is because instead of your body having to wear itself out and expend energy to digest and eliminate heavy, unnatural foods which in themselves contain little Life-Force, it now easily digests and absorbs foods which have much Life-Force in them. You cannot overeat fruits and vegetables if you do not use them in combination with undesirable foods.

Organically grown fruits and vegetables. There are two basic reasons for the devitalization of our food in America. One is the tampering with and alteration of it by human hands. The second is the longstanding use of improper fertilizers in the growing of it.

In our country most fertilizers are "inorganic"—that is, made from non-living (chemical) substances. Such fertilizers devitalize the plant foods to which they are applied.

One of the things that happens to any nutritive substance that enters a living organism is its being absorbed into the cells of the plant or animal. Whatever is absorbed into the cells of a living being becomes part of that plant or animal. Conversely, the plant or animal is affected by that substance and tends to manifest its characteristics.

Bodies are made of living, organic, chemical substances. When we feed bodies inorganic chemical substances, they become starved for the real sustainer of life—*Prana,* or Life-Force. When we feed plants—vegetables and fruits—inorganic food in the form of inorganic or chemically manufactured fertilizers, the plants become deficient in the Life-Force. When we then eat those plants for sustenance, we are feeding ourselves material that just does not give us life, that does not replenish our cells with living matter. We are starving ourselves.

No wonder America is so plagued with deficiency diseases. It is a tragic irony that the richest nation on earth suffers from diseases caused by improper eating and, actually, malnutrition.

If farmers replace inorganic fertilizers with organic fertilizers, that is, natural compost, made in the correct age-old way, it is our contention that our national disease rate would be considerably lowered. Compost is the correctly proportioned combination of dried and aged animal and plant manures. How simple the solution is, but how difficult to change from our present way.

In any case, you as an individual will be doing yourself the utmost good to seek out in your community a place where you can obtain fruits and vegetables grown organically.

Note: If you are seriously ill or under a physician's care, we recommend that you discuss any nutritional change you wish to make with him.

The Yogic concept of disease, however, differs from that of medical science. To the Yogi, all diseases can be prevented by proper care of the body, which includes, of course, proper nutrition. Immunity is something built up by the body itself if the body is given an unobstructed chance to do so. Immunity from disease is the body's natural state.

To the Yogi, germs are but carrion that multiply and thrive on an already diseased body. The true basic cause of disease is the improper functioning of the process of elimination. Internal purity —through correct circulation throughout the body and the natural condition of the internal organs—perfects the total process of elimination. Correct natural diet promotes internal cleanliness. This, plus the profound Yoga physical techniques, puts the body in such a condition that it becomes more and more free every day from disease.

The different diseases are but varying symptoms or manifestations of one cause. That cause is the imperfect elimination of toxic waste from the body.

By means of Yoga the lungs, kidneys, colon and skin perform their functions of elimination at top efficiency. By correct natural diet the cells are replenished with *living* material. The body rebuilds its natural immunity to the common diseases and infirmities of the human race.

Raw vegetable juices. The finest liquid you can put into your body is the juice of raw vegetables. It is water, but living, vital organic water, supplying you with minerals the quality of which cannot be excelled anywhere in all of nature. Raw vegetable juices are among the most sattvic of all foods. They cool, soothe and alkalize your body, counteracting in nature's perfect way the acid overbalance in the average person's system. The minerals and vitamins in raw vegetable juices are the most easily absorbed of all foods.

So wonderful for health are these juices that the correctly prescribed combinations of them have been known to cure the severest illnesses of man.

Some vegetables are very strong and have too sudden and powerful a cleansing effect upon the body. Among these are beets, cabbage, parsley and spinach. Small quantities of such strong vegetable juices have to be mixed with the more mild and sweet juices such as carrot and celery. Carrot juice is extremely mild and soothing and can be drunk to your heart's content.

Herb teas. Here is an unappreciated body of priceless knowledge. It is unfortunate how unaware America is of these venerable health-giving substances.

Herbs, taken in the form of tea, have great powers of regulating body functions. They are powerful therapeutic tonics.

The following herbs are highly recommended. They purify the blood, soothe the stomach and have an extremely regenerating effect upon the internal organs. Their specific effect can be found in any reputable book on herbs.

Red Clover	Camomile
Shave Grass	Watercress
Desert (Squaw) Grass	Peppermint
Alfalfa	

Full information on these wonderful plants is available in libraries and in bookstores specializing in health. Herbs have been used as the basis of an entire system of medicine in China for thousands of years, and the claims made for them are based on millions of case histories throughout the centuries, as well as modern observation and research.

Herb teas are simple to prepare but must be prepared correctly. Heat water until it begins to come to a heavy boil. Remove it from the flame and, just as the bubbles begin to subside, throw in a heaping tablespoon of herb (or the tea bag, if you obtain your herb in that form). Make sure all the herb material becomes soaked at once. Cover the container and allow the herb to steep in the hot water for at least three minutes. Strain and drink. Most people enjoy mixing the herb tea with some honey (tupelo honey is recommended) or molasses. If you prefer to use sugar as a sweetener, use raw unrefined sugar only.

Many people cultivate a taste for the straight herb tea. This is only a matter of personal preference.

Unless limited by prescription, you can drink herb tea at least as many times a day as you would drink regular tea or coffee. It is indeed the supreme replacement for tea or coffee, substituting the most healthful ingredients possible for those which are consistently harmful.

How Much to Eat

It is infinitely better to eat a small quantity of high-quality food than to eat a large quantity of poor-quality food.

It is neither healthy nor desirable to feel "stuffed" after a meal. The best state in which to get up from a meal is one of being not hungry any longer but not "full."

The quantity we are used to eating is only a habit, something we are conditioned to. After a short transition period you will become used to eating in moderate quantity, and you will feel wonderful—physically and mentally—by so doing.

Our three-meal-a-day habit is not dictated to us by the laws

of nature. On the contrary, we have allowed custom and the clock
to distort the laws of nature and our natural eating routine.

The Process of Eating

Do not think it an extreme statement when the Yogi states that
about one-third of the digestive process is supposed to take place
in the mouth.

The more food is chewed, the more efficiently can the digestive
juices of the stomach work upon the food. The more efficiently
the digestive juices of the stomach do their work on food, the
better prepared the food is for absorption when it reaches the
small intestine. Thus when you chew food properly the tissues
and the very cells of your body receive more nourishment, more
vitamins and essential minerals, ounce for ounce, than when
food is chewed in the usual way.

We Americans are as a group the worst offenders against
nature's laws and the health of our own bodies when it comes
to gulping our food.

The correct way to eat is to chew everything until it is a liquid
and then to swallow the liquid. Then swallow whatever solid
bulk is left. Mainly, as much as possible, liquefy your food in your
mouth. If this sounds extreme or peculiar, it is only because you
are not used to doing it. After a little while it becomes a habit
and you do it as naturally and unconsciously as you chew at
present.

By so chewing, you give the powerful and wonderful digestive
glands of the mouth ample time to mix their juices with the food.
Then, when the food reaches the stomach, the stomach and its
digestive glands do not have to do their own work *plus* the work
of the mouth and its glands.

Terrible diseases are generated and aided by the gulping habits
—ulcers, nervous stomach, colitis, indigestion, heartburn and
others.

By chewing correctly you get *more* nutritional value from eating as little as *half* your customary diet. You receive all the more

benefit on top of this if you alter your diet to accord with the natural food principle. Apply this technique of chewing as well as the use of natural foods for a few weeks and you will be amazed at the results.

Nourishment

We eat to gain that supreme universal force which we have translated as the Life-Force. We see then that there is more to eating than the taking in of a certain quantity of physical elements. Some foods give us greater access to *Prana*, or Life-Force. Other foods obstruct our access to this force.

The Life-Force available to us depends upon the condition of internal cleanliness of our bodies. The human body has very much the nature of a sponge. It is of the utmost importance to know *how well things flow through it*. The very choice of *what* is to enter the body is determined as much by how perfectly it will flush through the body as by what nutriments the material contains.

Three things can happen to whatever we eat.

1. Part of the food is absorbed into our blood stream and eventually reaches our cells and becomes part of us. Our entire being is then altered by the nature of such substances. We in time take on the qualities of what we eat.

2. Part of the food is expelled—from our skin, respiratory system, kidneys and colon—as waste.

3. Part of the food is neither absorbed to merge with our bodies nor is expelled as waste. This part becomes a sticky gluelike residue which lines our mucus membranes and clogs whatever space in our organism it can lodge in—the colon, the lungs, the sinuses, etc.

This is a new concept to most people. That is why the Yogi stresses the eating of foods which have the ability to cleanse the body, to flush through the spongelike structure of the body and even dissolve residues that have accumulated in the past. Fresh vegetables and fruits and their juices have the greatest power to do this. Citrus fruits are especially powerful cleansers. Strawberries and pineapples also perform this function. The papaya, one of nature's greatest gifts to man's health, is a superb cleanser, especially of the large intestine.

Just as a sponge must be kept clean so that whatever enters the network of passageways and openings of which it is composed can flow easily through it without clogging and filling it up with impurities, so must the human body be able to draw food substances through itself, absorbing what is needed and expelling perfectly all of the remainder.

Foods which form the sticky, unhealthy residual substance of which we spoke are refined flour products, all starches that have been tampered with by man, meat (especially in combination with starch), butter and other animal fats, and other food products which we shall enumerate later.

What is so important about keeping the body free of such residue? The Yogi tells us, from thousands of years of observation, experiment and experience, that an internally pure or clean body is resistant to disease and possesses as well much greater access to the vitality and energy provided by the Life-Force. Indeed, he tells us it is only when the passageways and tissues are obstructed with unnatural residues that disease can take hold of the organism, that the clogging of the body by impurities is *the* cause of disease. That is why we stress improvement and maintenance of proper circulation by the Yogic physical postures, the correct functioning of the organs of elimination by the cleansing techniques and the replacement of mucus-forming foods by cleansing foods.

The Yogi states that no germ can harm or multiply in or aid a diseased condition in a body that has sufficient cleanliness. This state of internal cleanliness is not difficult to attain, nor is it arrived at by some strange, extreme process. The simple application of the Yogic physical techniques and a diet changed to the natural food principle will immediately start the transformation.

Sattvic foods—natural organic fruits and vegetables—lighten the body, cleanse the internal organs and tissues and provide great energy by allowing the Life-Force to function freely through the body. These foods make you resistant to common diseases and increase the alertness and clarity of your mind. All of this results in an eventual expansion of consciousness and, if it is the individual's goal, the opportunity of experiencing one's original, or spiritual, nature. Thus profoundly, for positive or negative, can our diet and eating habits affect our lives.

Common Foods

Let us consider some of the foods which are thought of as basic in the average American's diet.

White sugar and white flour. White flour and white sugar do not exist in nature. Man created them. He took the brown or dark part out of flour and sugar, threw it aside and packaged the bleached remainder for human consumption. White flour and white sugar and all the products composed of them are among the most harmful foods you can put into your body.

There are two main reasons for this. First, the dark part—that which the manufacturers throw away—contains the vitamins and other nutritional elements. The white part by itself is little more than mere bulk which makes your body highly acid and at the same time clogs your system. Second, *nature puts into all its foods those chemical elements that digest each particular food in combination with the digestive fluids of your body.* When the brown part of the sugar plant, for example, is removed by man, your body must greatly increase its efforts to digest whatever minute nutriments are left in the material and to eliminate this white bulk. Thus instead of adding to your body, white sugar drains energy from your body by forcing the body itself to make up for what has been taken out of the sugar. The "energy" you get from white sugar is illusive. It is a temporary "hopping up" of your body. In the long run, refined sugar drains your Life-Force. Besides this, the eating of refined sugar becomes no different from an addiction. This applies to all white sugar products—cakes, candy, soft drinks, etc.

The same principle applies to bleached or refined flour. Thus white bread gives you nothing but dead bulk which eventually turns to a sticky pastelike substance in your body. This substance causes, in turn, a great strain upon your organs of digestion and elimination.

We cannot overemphasize the negative and even destructive effects of white sugar and white flour and products made from them.

It is simple to change this negative eating habit to a positive and healthy diet. Simply eat bread made from whole grain. Do not accept mixtures of white and whole grain flour. Such mixtures of quality do not work out. In most instances, if you mix good and bad, you do not get medium quality or average—you get bad. Make sure the bread you buy is whole grain and says so on the package without reservations—the darker the bread the better. Pumpernickel, one-hundred per cent stone ground whole wheat, whole grain rye bread; these are good. It is best if wheat is stone ground. Wheat is a very sensitive grain and easily destroyed nutritionally by overheating while being milled. Correct stone grinding avoids this.

As for sugar, the addiction which most people have to refined sugar is more difficult to break. So few products are made from natural whole sugar. You will probably have to go to a health food store to find such products. It is a good habit to frequent these stores. In the long run you save both money and your health.

For everyday sugar, use raw sugar—in general, the darker the better. For the cakes and candies you want, eat those made from raw natural whole sugar. Molasses and honey are the supreme substitutes for refined sugar. Besides the negative effects of refined sugar which we spoke of, there are the obvious well-known destructive results—decayed and eventually lost teeth, eruptions and negative conditions of the skin, and even certain major ailments.

Besides substituting for refined sugar, molasses and honey have positive healthful effects in themselves. They are most nourishing. Honey soothes the digestive tract, and certain kinds of honey even have a good effect upon the heart. Molasses is one of the finest and richest sources of iron, which purifies and improves the condition of the blood of your body. Molasses is that part of the cane sugar plant which is thrown away in the refining. Molasses puts iron into the blood. This iron draws increased amounts of oxygen into the blood stream from the air that is breathed into the lungs. This purifies and enriches the blood, increasing the Life-Force, so much of which is carried by the oxygen in our atmosphere. In turn it increases our natural energy and also increases our body's natural resistance to disease.

Meat. The eating of meat is an issue of great controversy. The viewpoints range from those who believe in strict vegetarianism to those who consider the consuming of meat an absolute necessity to life and health.

In the long run, those who advocate eating meat base their strongest argument on the nutritional value of the protein in meat. To this the vegetarians answer by saying that the protein of meat is of the lowest *quality* and that, ounce for ounce, your body receives more and better protein from certain cheeses, nuts and other non-flesh foods.

Those who do not believe in the eating of meat present further arguments in support of their point of view. Some of these are:

1. Certain creatures are meant by nature to be carnivorous. These creatures are identifiable by their teeth. Carnivorous animals—like the leopard, lion, tiger, dog, cat and crocodile—have sharp pointed teeth. Their teeth are designed to enable them to tear and chew meat.

Other creatures—such as the horse, cow and human beings— are constructed so that they can cut and grind plants with their teeth.

2. Tough, indigestible fibrous material in meat lodges in the colon and becomes the cause of negative conditions in that area.

3. Meat becomes highly toxic in the human system, especially when combined with certain other foods.

4. Meat, being extremely difficult to digest, causes overworking of the digestive glands and organs as well as overheating of the body.

Meat is highly rajasic in nature and perpetuates the cycle of excessive sensual attachment rather than normalizing and assuaging it.

5. Further technical argument presented by non-meat eaters deals with internal (intestinal) structure that differentiates carnivorous from herbivorous animals and places man further in the herbivorous category.

6. There is a physical, moral and spiritual degradation in the killing of animals for the purpose of eating their dead bodies.

Without a point-by-point agreement with these arguments, the Yogis do place themselves on the side of those who favor a non-meat diet. The Yogis further cite longstanding evidence that non-meat eaters, although perhaps not as strong (in the sense of being able to lift heavy objects) as meat eaters, nevertheless far exceed meat eaters when it comes to endurance and long-lasting energy.

The Yogis state that if the proper substitutes for the protein and other food elements in meat are eaten—such as nuts, cheese, avocado, etc.—the non-meat eater will have a cleaner, healthier and much more energetic physical organism than the meat eater and at the same time will have clearer and more alert senses and mind.

However, the principle of moderation is uppermost. You cannot hurry the results of this study. If you have been a steady meat eater all your life, we recommend a transition period in changing from a meat to a non-meat diet. And remember that meat substitutes must be used on a comparative quantity basis. A few nuts and two or three ounces of cheese will not suffice for a person who has been accustomed to eating a pound of steak at a time.

The benefits of a non-meat diet are:

Physically:
a) better digestion

b) cleaner body
c) more energy
d) greater endurance
e) a lighter, more "alive" feeling
f) healthier digestive tract and internal organs
g) calmer nerves

Mentally:
a) sharper senses
b) more alert mind
c) less sleep needed
d) a calmer, less agitated mind

Spiritually:
a) a disassociation from the slaughter of animals
b) the elevation that automatically occurs with the ceasing of eating dead bodies
c) the unfolding of sattvic traits of character
d) greater facility on the path of spiritual enlightenment

Poultry. Most poultry raised in the United States now is fed a semi-artificial diet which makes it reach a full physical size in an unnaturally accelerated time. The flesh of these creatures is deficient in nutritional elements compared to a fowl fed in the natural manner and allowed to mature at a normal rate.

Besides this general lack of nutritional value, most of the principles which spoke against the eating of meat in general apply to chicken and other fowl.

Fish. Fish possess qualities that may stand in favor of their consumption by humans. But much depends on the way in which they are prepared.

Fish contain many nutritional elements not as easily obtained elsewhere by the average person. They contain minerals that are body-building and aid in the normal functioning of the glands, especially the thyroid gland.

Fish contain iodine, potassium, phosphorus and other vital elements.

They are best eaten in a broth. Make sure you drink all the liquid of the broth. Broiled and baked fish are acceptable. Frying is harmful. Small quantities of fish eaten raw and chewed well will give you the minerals and nutriments it contains.

The approval of eating fish, correctly prepared, of course, may seem a departure from the tradition of Yoga. It is, however, taken here in respect to two factors:

1. We live in a temperate country, many parts of which have a hard, even severe, winter. It is more important to obtain vital nutriments to maintain health than to adhere to an abstract, no matter how perfect, principle. In consideration of the dire necessity of bolstering our nation's declining health, Yoga must remain pre-eminently a practical science and not a small extremist cult.

2. The principle of common-sense moderation must hold itself forth, especially when dealing with a practical, down-to-earth people such as Americans. It is more important for a person used to eating flesh for a lifetime to practice some Yoga than to cease practicing through discouragement due to inability to adhere to the highest absolute principles of purity. Yoga is for people. Eating fish is a good aid in the transition from a meat diet to the more desirable and ultimately more healthy non-meat diet.

It is better to practice some Yoga than none, for the benefits of a moderate practice of Yoga are great.

Dairy foods. The true worth of dairy foods in America is deceptive. Most people, upon first eliminating meat from their diets, look to dairy foods to replace the protein provided by meat. They forget that dairy foods come in different qualities, some being natural and more healthful than others.

In the realm of dairy products, as a substitute for meat protein, the best foods are cottage cheese, farmer cheese and fresh, unaged Wisconsin cheeses.

Aged and sharp cheeses contain chemical products of their fermentation which render them unwholesome. A higher quality calcium, more easily digested and absorbed, is also obtained from the cottage and fresh cheeses. Yogurt is a food highly beneficial for the colon.

Skim or non-fat milk is in our opinion far superior to regular pasteurized or homogenized milk. Whole milk is, if course, the best quality milk, but it is difficult to obtain and in some states is even outlawed. Pasteurization kills the living organic part of milk and leaves a dead, highly mucus-forming food very much devoid of its original natural good qualities. The advertisement of milk as a perfect or complete food applies to whole milk, not to the dead pasteurized product.

We believe that the substitution of fresh raw carrot juice, for example, in place of a considerable part of the heavy pasteurized milk diet that is forced on children, would result in less susceptibility to colds.

Most cheeses are also pasteurized or processed unnaturally these days, and so it is difficult to obtain dairy products in their best state. But you must do as well as you can. Cottage and fresh Wisconsin cheeses are good. Farmer cheese and Italian Ricotta cheese are even better.

If you can obtain goat's milk in your community, do not be afraid to pay the higher price per quart for it. In the long run you will save money, while benefiting your health immeasurably. Goat's milk is far more suitable for human use than cow's milk and is highly recommended. A small amount of it goes a long way toward providing the finest quality calcium and other nutriments needed by your body.

We have already said much about protein. Let us conclude this subject by stating that a small quantity of high-quality, easily absorbed protein is far preferable to a large quantity of low-quality protein as is customarily available in meat and tampered foods.

Artificial Stimulants

Under this heading we will include alcohol, tobacco, condiments, artificial preservatives, coffee and tea.

Alcohol. Alcohol is the most tamasic (density producing) of all foods. It is a medicine. The comical phrase applied to alcoholic beverages, "for medicinal purposes only," should in reality be adhered to. It fogs the mind, distorts the passions and feelings, deranges the senses and, with prolonged use, destroys the human body. But if you do take a drink *occasionally* and know that you will always be so inclined, do *not* feel guilty because of it. The practice of your physical Yoga techniques and eating correctly will far and away offset the effects of a genuinely occasional drink.

Tobacco. Smoking is extremely bad for you, despite advertisements and propaganda which imply that it is not injurious. Smoking definitely contributes to the incidence of lung cancer. It is an irritant to the membrane lining the throat, bronchial passages and lungs. Rather than steadying the nerves, it does the opposite, having a destructive effect upon the nervous system. The coal tars carried by the fumes adhere to the sticky tissue of the lungs and in short order impair the functioning of the lungs, interfering with the process of oxygen absorption and causing shortness of breath, lack of endurance, harmful coughs and other negative effects.

There is much discussion nowadays of the deeper psychological reasons behind the smoking habit. There is an element of truth in these reasons, but many people use them as an excuse for their inability to successfully break the smoking habit. No matter how difficult it is to break the smoking habit, the structure and cure of the habit is not as complex and awesome as psychologists claim. Once again the Yogi overcomes a serious negative condition by the application of internal cleanliness.

Whoever correctly practices the Yoga breathing technique which cleanses the lung tissue of accumulated coal tars and other impurities will find the desire and need to smoke diminished in a manner corresponding to the sincerity of his effort. Pure lung tissue will not accept tobacco fumes, and the individual in a state of cleanliness will find himself unable to enjoy or even tolerate smoking any longer.

The general bodily cleanliness induced by eating according to the natural food principle aids very much in the overcoming of this harmful, unhealthy habit. Smoking definitely decreases one's access to the Life-Force.

Condiments. Spices are rajasic foods. They heat the body and lead us away from control of our senses and mind. They serve no positive purpose beyond the titillation of our sense of taste. The more we use spices for flavoring, the less can we taste the actual and delicious flavor of man's natural foods. Food can be deliciously flavored by the use of natural foods and juices, onions, garlic, green peppers, tomatoes, etc.

Salt is a necessity. Vegetable salt and natural sea salt are the best kinds to use. It is worth a few cents a pound more to get these kinds of easily digestible salts rather than settle for the average "iodized" commercial brands.

It may seem that spices belong to the category of natural foods and should therefore be altogether positive, but when you consider their agitating effect upon the body it becomes apparent that this is not true.

Artificial preservatives. We speak here of such things as the use of sodium glutinate to retard spoilage of bread and sulfur dioxide to preserve dried fruits. The Yogi classifies such chemicals as impurities and advises against their use. In this instance you may have to hunt around a little to find bread or dried fruits and other products without these preservatives in them, but once you go to this trouble the result is most worth-while. You have only one body for this lifetime, and the keeping of that body in a healthy state is well worth a little initial effort. Once again, you would do well to check with your local health food store for breads, dried fruits and other food products made without preservatives.

Coffee. Coffee contains caffeine, which is a poison and which has a negative effect upon the nervous system. The stimulation that one feels after drinking one or two cups of coffee is a false energy. The caffeine shocks the nervous system, producing an illusory awakening. Actually, practice of Yogic breathing techniques will awaken, clarify and alert your mind far beyond the degree that coffee can. If you can alter your diet away from the body- and mind-burdening foods and toward the natural food principle, you will experience an awakening and clarity of your mental faculties and a physical energy that far surpass the effects of any stimulants. The so-called energy produced by coffee is temporary. It leads to a dependency on the stimulant, an addiction, the well-known "coffee habit." The resulting energy that comes from the eating of natural foods is cumulative and long-lasting.

To offset the acquired enjoyment of the taste and custom of drinking coffee, there are a number of coffee substitutes available. These are made of cereal and have a taste so similar to coffee that you need not be deprived of the pleasure of hot beverages of that type.

Tea. Tea contains tannic acid. This too cannot be considered a good thing to put into your organism.

Both the coffee and tea habits can be turned to your advantage by the substituting of herb teas in their place.

Combinations

The subject of what foods to eat in combination is of utmost importance. You can waste a considerable part of your time, effort and money when you begin altering your diet to the wrong combinations.

A fundamental principle to always keep in mind is:

Eat as few different kinds of food as you can at each meal without making the meal unpleasant or unnutritive.

With this in mind, we will list the most common bad food combinations.

Meat and starch. If you do eat meat, at least don't combine it with starch, such as potatoes or bread. This combination is highly acid-forming, fattening and, with prolonged use, results in negative conditions of the nerves and the kidneys.

Coffee and cream. The combination of cream in coffee is also highly acid-forming and is bad for the complexion.

Sweet and acid fruits. If you are on the pure diet and are subsequently using fresh fruits as one of your mainstays, do not mix sweet fruits—pear, plum, apple, peach, banana, papaya, etc.— with the so-called acid fruits—lemon, lime, orange, grapefruit, strawberry, pineapple—at the same sitting. They cancel out much of the tremendous cleansing value to be had from each when eaten separately. Wait fifteen or twenty minutes between eating these two types of fruit.

Liquids and solids. Beverages should be drunk before a meal. Liquids go through an empty stomach very quickly, and the relief from thirst or the nutriments needed in liquid form are obtained thusly.

But if you mix liquid with the solid foods that you eat at a meal, the digestive juices have a considerably more difficult time digesting the material in the stomach and preparing it for absorption in the small intestine.

Adhering to the same principle, you should not drink for a half hour or so after eating.

Supplements

Considering the devitalized nature of most foods in our country, due to inorganic fertilizers, improper irrigation, canning, freezing, etc., supplements are recommended as being necessary.

Beware of eccentric fads, but use the necessary basic supplements to make your nutritional intake complete.

A good high-potency multi-vitamin is basic, either in tablet or liquid form. Organic vitamins are better than those made from coal tar derivative and other inorganic chemical sources. Organic vitamins take a little longer to begin doing their work, but the effect is longer-lasting and much more genuinely therapeutic.

Two vitamins which people have an especially hard time providing themselves with are the B-Complex group and vitamin C. Neither vitamin B1 nor vitamin C are stored for long in the body. They must be replenished continually. Extra vitamin B1 (and the B-Complex group) and vitamin C can be well used by many people, even beyond the amounts provided by the average multivitamin formula.

Other beneficial supplements are as follows:

Raw wheat germ (rich in vitamin B1)

Wheat germ oil (a fine source of vitamin E)

Unsulphured molasses (one of the best sources of iron)
Lecithin (good for the nerves)
Concentrated sea water (splendid source of minerals)
Protein (in powder or tablet form)
Amino acids (in powder or tablet form)
Most of these foods can be obtained at your local health food store.

Your Taste Preference

Some people say that vegetables and salads and other natural foods taste too bland for them and that they crave the taste pleasure which they obtained from their previous diet.

This is only a temporary transitional phase in the *development* of the sense of taste. Actually, a meat and artificially flavored diet blunts the taste. Only when you have eliminated false condiments and bad combinations from your diet will you be able to truly start "tasting."

The vegetables that may seem bland to you at first will undergo a great taste change in time. Your jaded taste buds will become purified and will retain their natural sensitivity. Then you will truly taste the delicious character of foods as they were meant to be enjoyed by man.

Fasting

Fasting is the most ancient and perfect method known to man of reconditioning, purifying and curing the body. It is strange how few people know the exact method of this wonderful system of self-therapy.

When animals are hurt or sick, they fast to heal themselves. There is a part of them that knows by instinct that the temporary stopping of the intake of food enables the body to cleanse, rebuild and heal itself. Man has lost this instinctive wisdom and must relearn it.

The fasting itself is easy. The secret lies in correctly *beginning* and especially in correctly *breaking* the fast.

1. The Fruit Fast. This consists of eating only fresh fruits, in proper combination, for the duration of your fast.

2. The Mono-Diet Fruit Fast. This consists of eating only *one* kind of fruit at a sitting for a meal or for a day. For example, a breakfast of only fresh cherries, a lunch of peaches, etc.

3. The Juice or Liquid Fast. This consists of drinking only fresh fruit juices during the period of the fast. This is the strongest of the three partial fasts and has powerful cleansing and healing effects.

4. The Complete Fast. This consists of eating nothing at all during the fasting period and only drinking water when thirsty. (During a complete fast water is to be drunk only when *thirsty* and not as an attempt to assuage any feelings of hunger.)

Beginning the fast. The last meal you eat before beginning a fast has considerable effect upon the fast. It should be an evening meal and should consist of nourishing but easily digested and *easily eliminated* food. The best type of final hot meal before a fast is correctly cooked (that is, lightly or moderately steamed) fresh vegetables. By having a cleansing effect in itself, however mild, this meal will prepare you for the fast.

During the fast. The noticeable effects upon you depend, of course, upon the length of your fast. The symptoms are usually the same for any of the first three days. Due to the profound cleansing effect of this process, toxins are drawn from the tissues and brought into the blood stream to be expelled from the body. During these periods a person may feel headaches or physical weakness. These intervals are short. The best way to deal with them is to rest completely and to passively allow the deep cleansing process to occur.

Many people feel no negative symptoms but are instead full of energy.

Throughout nearly any fasting period, the intervals of fatigue alternate with periods of abundant energy. This has to do with the rhythm of toxins entering and leaving the bloodstream as well as other physiological factors.

Breaking the fast. This is the key to a successful fast. By breaking the fast incorrectly you will negate most of the good it would have done for your body and mind, and in some instances you could even hurt yourself.

Fasts must be broken in the following manner:

Break a fast in the morning. First drink a glass of freshly squeezed fruit juice of a cleansing or a mildly laxative nature. Orange, grapefruit, prune, fig or genuine grape juice are recommended. If you have fasted for more than three days, we suggest diluting the juice with half pure (spring or distilled, not tap) water.

Wait fifteen or twenty minutes, and then eat a breakfast of fresh fruits alone. Eat as much as you desire, but do not allow your mind to overrule your body in dictating the quantity.

For lunch and dinner of that first day eat as strictly according to the natural food principle as you can, taking care to not eat anything heavy or pasty. It would be well for the dinner of that first day of breaking the fast to be another meal of cooked fresh vegetables.

Breaking the fast carefully in this manner will ensure that the cleansing process of fasting takes place completely. Recall the image used earlier where the body is described as having the nature of a sponge. This image applies to the fast. The period of fasting corresponds to the sponge being squeezed and the impure materials being eliminated from its deep recesses. The application of food to the body after the fast corresponds to fresh, clean water being sucked into the sponge after squeezing. If you squeeze the dirty water out of a sponge and replace it with pure water enough times, eventually the sponge will be clean all the way through. That is what fasting does. And that is why it is necessary to supply the body with pure, highly nourishing and cleansing foods after any fast.

Please bear in mind that at least two days of "recuperation" should be allowed immediately after a fast for every day of fasting.

When to fast and for how long. We do not recommend prolonged fasts unless prescribed by and overseen by a qualified physician or qualified reputable expert in the field. Neither do we recommend a prolonged fast for anyone who has not, with moderate Yoga practice and periodic short fasts, prepared his body for the extreme cleansing effect of a longer fast.

We recommend that the following moderate practice of fasting be attempted by anyone interested in the rejuvenation of the internal tissues, glands and organs. Fast one day each second week, partially or completely, for a period of six months. After that you may, if you are so inclined, fast one day each week in the same manner. We recommend beginning with the fruit fast, going on to the juice fast for several times and then fasting that one day completely.

The higher implications of fasting. Besides cleansing, healing, rejuvenating and rendering the body more resistant to common ailments, fasting has a deeper significance. All spiritual leaders of the human race have either practiced fasting or recommended its use. Jesus Christ, Buddha, Mohammed, Moses, the Enlightened Sages of China, Japan and India—all have fasted or taught its use.

When the body is not taking in food the following happens:

1. The internal organs rest and by resting regenerate themselves.

2. The body is cleansed of accumulated impurities and attains a more sattvic state.

3. Unburdened by the denser form of nourishment, the body increases its intake of and subsists more directly on the more subtle and primary nourishment, namely *Prana,* or Life-Force.

4. Despite early negative symptoms in some instances, the mind is cleared, the individual consciousness is expanded and the individual gains a wider and more universal insight into the nature of the self and the world.

5. Actual spiritual insight and experience are to be had when one goes through a complete fast for the ultimate length of time necessary to his organism. This—only after complete long-term preparation—can range anywhere from thirty to ninety days, depending on all the complex factors involved.

The attainment of complete or intense spiritual experience

through long fasting is a subject of supreme importance. This present book is not the place to enter it. Suffice it to say that this claim for the extreme prolonged fast is true but must not be attempted without expert supervision and under correct conditions.

Here is summarization by example of the recommended short (partial or complete) fast for health. If you wanted to fast, let us say, on a Saturday, a one-day fast, you would proceed as follows: On Friday evening you would eat a dinner of cooked fresh vegetables. After this you would eat nothing—or subsist on fruit juices if you were on a liquid fast—the rest of Friday evening and night and nothing on Saturday. On Sunday morning you would break the fast in the prescribed manner. You would attempt to adhere to the natural food principle as much as possible for the next two days.

Sample Menus

The Yogi advocates no "diet" as such nor any crash weight reducing program nor the present fad of calorie counting. All such practices have temporary and futile results. The Yogi teaches the *basic principles* of nutrition and offers a general formula within the framework of which an individual may satisfy his taste preferences as well as his need to look, feel and be healthy and in top shape.

Here is one general sample formula which you can use as a ready reference.

In Yogi there is no place for guilt. So-called backsliding is not backsliding to the Yogi but merely a law of progress in learning. No one progresses in a straight line but rather in a series of steps forward and then a lesser number of steps back, then forward, then back a little, etc.

There must be no psychological pressure on "forcing" in this program to attain the highest peak of lifelong health and well-being. If you are ever seized by a craving to eat a hot fudge sundae or a big steak, by all means go ahead and do so and be glad of it. Then resume your correct eating on good terms and as friend to Yoga and to yourself.

BREAKFAST

A glass of fresh fruit juice.
Orange, fig, prune, grapefruit, grape or apple juice. As large a glass as you desire.

Wait five or ten minutes before eating the rest of your breakfast.
Cereal
Whole grain cereal only.
Hot cereal in cold weather. Cold cereal in hot weather.
Add a generous helping of raw wheat germ to the cereal.
You may add fresh fruit to your cereal if you wish.

or

Fruit
A bowl of fresh fruit in season.

or

Yogurt
Plain or with a generous helping of raw wheat germ and raw honey (preferably Tupelo honey).
Yogurt also mixes well with fresh sweet fruit.
Herb Tea
Plain or flavored with molasses or honey as you prefer.

LUNCH

Soup
Lima bean, vegetable, lentil, black bean, potato, split pea, onion, fish broth (never canned or frozen).
Soup is optional depending on your appetite.
It is best to drink soup ten minutes or so before eating the rest of your lunch.
Salad
Vegetable (raw always).
Suggested ingredients (choose two to four according to your taste preference):

Carrots, celery (chopped or stalk), onion, corn (yes, raw corn), lettuce, tomato, ripe olives, watercress, green peppers, cucumbers, radishes, cabbage, cauliflower.

Dressing: Safflower seed oil, soya oil, corn oil with or without lemon.

Cottage or farmer cheese mixes well with a fresh vegetable salad.

or

Fruit

Peaches, apples, plums, pears, bananas or any fresh fruit in season. Papaya is a marvelously therapeutic food when exactly ripe. Avocado, extremely high in protein, stuffed with cottage cheese.

If you have not eaten a fruit salad at breakfast, a fresh fruit salad for lunch is especially cooling in the summer.

Dried Fruits

Raisins, figs, prunes, dates, apricots, etc. These can be mixed in with a fresh sweet fruit salad.

They are splendid as a side dish.

Nuts

Brazil, walnut, pecan, cashew (unroasted and unsalted). This also as a side dish.

These mix well with dried fruits.

Cheese

If you have not mixed cottage or farmer cheese with your salad, some fresh Wisconsin cheese or Swiss cheese goes very well with this lunch.

Bread

You may eat one or two slices of genuine whole grain bread, according to your appetite.

Dessert

Pudding (brown rice pudding, for example).

or

Custard, made from low fat milk.

Gelatin.

or

Herb tea

Plain or with molasses or honey. Drink this as long *after* your lunch as possible.

Note: The above is a general reference list of those foods from which you can make a pure and very nourishing lunch. Apply it according to your needs.

If your basic lunch would consist of, for example, soup, vegetable salad and herb tea, you can satisfy your body's nutritional requirements and hunger by the nuts, dried fruits, cheese, bread and dessert. Thus does this general formula apply to those whose type of work or activity gives them a large or small appetite.

DINNER

Soup

The same as recommended for lunch.

Soup for dinner depends on your preference and appetite and not on whether or not you had some for lunch.

Fish

Lightly steamed, broiled or baked (never fried). Serve with one or two cooked vegetables. Avoid shell-fish.

or

Organ Meat

Liver, kidney, etc. Broiled and rare. Also served with cooked vegetables.

or

Cooked Vegetables

Carrots, onions, spinach, beets with their tops, corn, green peas, string beans. Lightly steamed so they still retain a crunchy freshness. Never overcook. Do not throw away the juice produced in their cooking but serve it to be drunk, for it is full of nutriments. Also baked potato, sweet potato, and baked eggplant.

Spaghetti

Or other similar starch product only if made of whole grain. These can be obtained in your local health food store.

Lettuce and Tomato Salad

As a suggested side dish.

Dessert
See Lunch.
Herb Tea
Same as lunch and breakfast.
Snacks
If you desire a snack between meals, you may indulge freely in nuts, dried fruits or a piece of raw fresh vegetable such as a carrot or a stalk of celery.
Raw Vegetable Juices
May be drunk at any time of the day except during meals or within an hour after eating.

Conclusion

Health, youth, endurance, energy, tranquility—these qualities and all qualities like them are the "normal" states of man. They are your birthright. All negative conditions, disease, infirmity, weakness, chronic fatigue, nervousness and the symptoms of old age are unnatural. These are imposed upon us and are departures from our true natural condition.

The function of eating correctly is to keep the Life-Force functioning freely and unobstructedly in and through us. This also is a primary purpose of the physical techniques. When we have full natural access to the great universal Life-Force, glowing good health is but a normal by-product.

Energy, like peace, is within you. The work of Yoga is simply to remove obstructions to the functioning of the natural forces that lie dormant within us.

Apply these wonderful vital Yoga techniques and the natural food principle to your life, be quietly diligent in this work, and you will enjoy the blessings of lifelong health and peace.

PART THREE
RAJA (MENTAL) YOGA

RAJA YOGA: THE SCIENCE
OF MIND CONTROL

Raja Yoga is the name given to the science, perfected thousands of years ago in India, of quieting and controlling the mind. It is practiced to attain real and lasting peace.

The method is called meditation, and that is the name we shall use interchangeably with the name Raja Yoga from now on. Meditation is a *simple, natural* process, and it is practiced in the same methodical step-by-step manner as are the physical techniques of Yoga.

Meditation is completely enjoyable and has the following results:

1. Relaxing the nervous system
2. Overcoming negative mental states such as anxiety, fear, anger, etc.
3. Increasing emotional control
4. Calming and quieting the mind
5. Providing the sincere practicer with a direct insight into the nature of his or her own self

People in all walks of life and in all parts of the world have practiced meditation for thousands of years. They have all attested to the same wonderful results.

Americans are very much in need of this science. We live at a pace that kills, and at the same time we are subjected to the most serious mental anxieties. Some of our pressures and anxieties are the same as those which people had thousands of years ago—money, domestic difficulties, problems of health, false notions of insecurity, and the dozens of problems, disappointments and frus-

155

trations that must be coped with every day. Other emotional mental and nervous pressures that we have are unique to our age; for example, the now nearly chronic dread of atomic war.

The need for meditation—a practical and efficient method of attaining peace of mind—is universal. We in America, especially, need this knowledge.

Meditation must be practiced. All the talking about it, studying about it or thinking *about* it that you can do will produce no results. Theorizing is worth absolutely nothing in this study. You must practice Yoga and know it by experience. In fact, the less you theorize about Yoga, to yourself as well as to others, the more successful will your practice be.

Raja Yoga (meditation) is simple, delightful and extremely rewarding in terms of tranquility, balance and clarity of mind. You will verify these claims if you apply yourself sincerely to the techniques taught in this book.

In this section on Raja Yoga, you will learn five major meditation (mental) techniques. There is no mystery or hocus-pocus about this simple science. Meditation is for anyone who will practice it. It does not clash with any person's background or belief. With it you can join the countless hundreds of thousands of people who have, through all ages and in all parts of the world, found harmony and inner peace by this means.

Yoga Is Neither Hypnosis nor Autosuggestion

Raja Yoga has no relation to hypnosis. On the contrary, meditation is *the* method known to man that counteracts the universal hypnotic state in which everyone lives.

We are hypnotized by our desires and by the objects of our desires and by a horde of illusory ideas and notions. Meditation is a way of *awakening* from the hypnotic states into which the "ten thousand things" of life have lured us.

Meditation Posture

In order to meditate you must sit in the correct position or meditation posture. This correct meditation posture is as follows:

1. Sit crosslegged on the floor.

You may use either of the three Yogi sitting postures, the SIMPLE POSTURE (see Figure 50), the HALF LOTUS (see Figure 52) or the FULL LOTUS (see Figure 54). Use whichever of these is the most comfortable for you.

2. Sit erectly.

In order to sit correctly, be sure that your nose is directly above your navel and that your ears are directly on a line above your shoulders.

Rest your wrists comfortably on your knees and keep your fingers in the position indicated in Figure 50.

When you sit erectly in this manner, your lungs are free to function to their full natural capacity and your heart and internal organs are not cramped.

Many people ask: "Why can't I practice meditation sitting in a chair or leaning back against a support or even lying down in greater comfort?"

The answer is that if you are more limp than in the correct, classic meditation posture, your self control tends to slip away easily. Your mind will soon wander, and you will become sleepy. This classic meditation posture has been used for thousands of years because it contributes most efficiently to the desired results. Your back muscles quickly become used to this way of sitting and are strengthened by it.

I recommend that you reread the discussion of benefits of the Yogic sitting positions in the physical section. Of course, if there is some physical reason why you cannot sit in the Yogic way—previous injury, etc.—then you may alter the posture to suit your condition.

Active and Passive Meditation

Meditation can be classified into two types: active and passive.

Active meditation consists of the mental techniques which you can practice in the midst of everyday action, while walking, riding, waiting and even in the act of business or communication.

Passive meditation is the type we are presently describing. It is the ancient classic method of sitting meditation. It consists of stilling the runaway mind in a quiet, unmoving manner.

Techniques of active meditation will be described under that heading.

Sitting Still

The first step in meditation consists of the preparation for meditating. This should be a methodical workout period in Hatha Yoga (following the practice schedules given in this book) ending with the ALTERNATE NOSTRIL BREATHING.

The second step is the assuming of the correct meditation posture.

The third step should be sitting still. This may sound ridiculously simple, but most people never sit still—not for as long as one minute—from one year to the next. So after assuming the correct meditation sitting posture (we will presume that your breath has been regulated to a long, even, quiet flow by the ALTERNATE NOSTRIL BREATHING), you must begin to be as absolutely unmoving as possible. Don't fidget. Don't shift about. Don't adjust yourself. Only the parts of your body involved in the breathing process should be moving in the correct free and relaxed manner. Blink normally of course. But besides these necessary functions, be as still as a statue.

Stillness

Stillness is a beautiful as well as a necessary thing. Especially in the confused hectic life we lead, we must practice stillness. Stillness is essential to success in passive meditation.

Your body and mind are in reality one thing, not two separate entities. What happens to your body happens to your mind. When your body moves, your mind moves correspondingly. When your body is agitated, nervous and fidgety, your mind will be similarly restless.

When you practice passive (sitting) meditation, keeping your body still and your breath quiet, long and even, your mind can and will begin to become quiet and unmoving.

A Basic Principle of Raja Yoga

Your mind is not "nothing" simply because you cannot see it with your eyes or experience it with any other of your senses. Your mind is made of something. It has a substance.

The substance of which your mind is made is refined indeed. Yet that organization of forces is material or substantial enough to be a super-efficient computing and tabulating machine and substantial enough to directly affect the material world around you.

The mind-substance is continually moving. So long as your mind moves without control, you can have no peace. So long as you are carried along helplessly by the movement and subsequent illusions of your everyday mind, you can never know who you really are nor can you ever experience life as it really is. (See *The Nature of the Mind.*) Reality, or the true nature of the world, is distorted as it filters through the uncontrolled movements of the mechanical mind.

As you cannot see through turbulent water, so can you not see through the movements of your mind-substance. But once movement is stilled, then you can see into and through your mind and experience your true original nature, learning by direct experience once and for all time who you are.

Concentration

Once you are sitting still and breathing quiet, complete breaths and are in the correct meditation posture, you can begin meditation.

It is necessary to be able to concentrate your attention upon one point before you can meditate. We are accustomed to spreading our minds upon the outside world according to how many of the "things" of the world around us lure or demand our attention. We are also used to a lifetime of allowing nearly every daydream to distract us and to prevent us from experiencing the living moment of reality.

The following is a thoroughly delightful exercise which will develop your ability to concentrate, or hold your mind on one point. Practice it every day, according to instructions.

Meditation Technique No. 1: Candle Concentration

This must be performed in a dark room.

Sit on the floor.

Place a lighted candle about an arm's length in front of you.

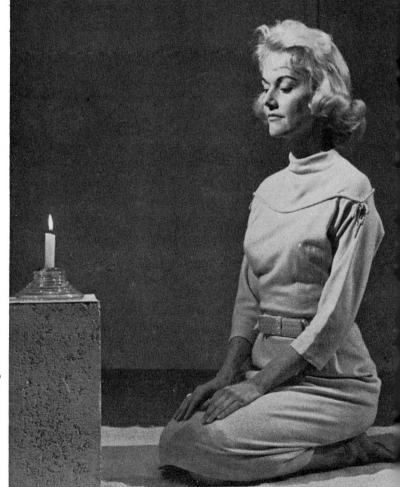

Figure 79

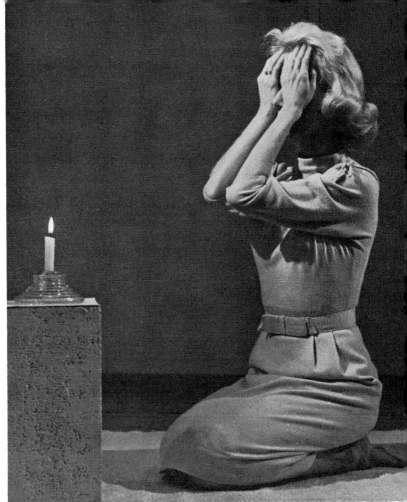

Figure 80

(Try to avoid having any draft touch the candle flame. That will make it waver, and it is best if the flame rises up straight and steady.)

Now gaze fixedly at the candle flame. Blink normally but keep your attention upon the flame. Do not look away from the flame even for a split second, and try not to allow your mind to wander elsewhere.

Concentrate your sight in this manner for three minutes. Your estimate of this time length will be sufficient and will become extremely accurate as the days progress.

Then take your hands and cup them over your *open* eyes. (Figure 80.)

Looking into the darkness of your cupped hands, you will see the after-image of the candle flame. The purpose of this exercise

161

is for you to keep that after-image in sight as long as you possibly can and to keep it steady in the center of your vision. Try not to let it waver or move about. If it recedes or fades out of sight, attempt to bring it back into view.

Practice this second part of the CANDLE CONCENTRATION technique for three minutes, the same length of time that you originally gazed at the actual flame. With this technique you will train your mind not to wander, to obey you and to be able to hold itself on one point, without which skills there can be no success in meditation.

Concentration and Discipline

Just as with the word "discipline," the word "concentration" seems to denote something unpleasant to the average person. Upon hearing these two words one usually thinks of a great strain, something involving tremendous effort of the will and mental faculties. This is a false impression, and the very first practice of Yoga proves it to be false.

Hatha Yoga, for example, is a discipline—indeed, one of the highest forms of self-discipline. Yet it is utterly enjoyable from the very beginning. In Hatha Yoga, you discipline what has been in nearly all cases a badly spoiled body, and instead of feeling any strain or effort of discipline, you feel the joy of total improvement and the release from the bondage of unnatural tension. Thus we see the true nature of self-discipline—that it is one of the highest pleasures and leads to the highest good.

Concentration in Raja Yoga is that self-discipline applied to the mind. The results correspond to those of Hatha Yoga. There is the fascinating exploration into your self. In the CANDLE CONCENTRATION technique your mind and nerves are relieved of tension. We will speak of further results of meditation under a later heading.

Meditation With and Without an Object

We have spoken of two kinds of meditation—active and passive. This division was based on the outward aspects of meditation;

that is, whether you are engaged in physical action during the time of meditation or whether you are sitting still.

There is another, and in a sense deeper, division of meditation. This consists of whether the student is meditating with an object or without an object.

Meditation with an object means that there is something *upon which* the person is meditating, upon which his mind is focused. This can be an object in the external world such as the candle in the technique you have just learned. It can be a religious image, a purely aesthetic (non-religious) work of art, or an object or scene of beauty from the world of nature. The object can also be internal, one formed in the mind, such as a picture image, a word, a phrase or a concept.

Meditation without an object is a higher, purer form of meditation. Indeed, meditation with an object can be considered to be a preparation for pure or non-objective meditation. Though the results of meditation with an object are great, the object in the mind is still an obstruction to the final goal of mental Yoga.

You must learn what Raja Yoga is by practicing a number of its forms. It is important and advisable for you to have the experience of meditation with an object before you go into objectless meditation.

About Withdrawal

Withdrawal is the temporary divorcement of yourself from the objects of the world around you that continually demand the attention of your mind and senses. There is a time to cater to the world around you and to the demands of your senses, and there is a time to put these things aside—in their place, so to speak— and proceed systematically with your journey toward the discovery of your real or intrinsic nature. The truth, as all sages in all lands have stated, is *within* you.

When the time comes to not pay Caesar, then let us not pay him. There is a time when you stop giving a spoiled child the attention he is demanding. Thus it is with the world around you. Once a day say to it, "you have had sufficient dominion over me

for now." Once a day, at least, you must assert your independence
from the hypnotic allure and from the continual empty promises
of the world. This is the time of withdrawal.

It is more than your right to temporarily withdraw. It is your
duty. And by so doing you return refreshed to the everyday
world and its responsibilities, enriched by the insight gained
through the practice of Yoga and fortified by your rest from the
constant tyranny of your senses and mind.

The Use of the Eyes in Meditation

All meditation, whatever technique you happen to be using
at the time, is a temporary withdrawal.

This is facilitated by one main technique employed in all meditation except when you use as your object something physical in
the external world. This technique is the correct use of your eyes
during meditation.

When practicing passive (sitting) meditation, focus your eyes
in toward you so that they gaze at or near the tip of your nose.

A good way to begin this is as follows: Hold your index finger
up about eight inches in front of your eyes. Focus your eyes at the
tip of it.

Now quickly take your finger away, but keep your eyes focused
where they were. When you do this, everything around you will
be blurred. With your eyes focused at this distance, there should
be no muscular strain. This blurring out of the objective world
around you is a pleasant sensation and is extremely restful for
your nervous system.

You may then practice bringing the focal point of your sight
in closer to the tip of your nose. *If you feel any strain or discomfort whatever in your eyes, do not focus them that closely toward
your nose.*

This discomfort means that your eye muscles are not used to
this position. As long as the outside world is blurred, you are
accomplishing the right thing with your eyes.

Each separate form in the objective world is crying out for your attention. Now you are asserting independence and mastery over your senses and their objects. The rewards are great indeed.

With a little practice your eyes will grow accustomed to this position. Do not force them into it.

Attempt to keep your sight on the center line that separates the right side from the left side of your nose. It is quite like a game. Do not allow your sight to slip over to the right or left. Be gentle. In time your gaze will become steady. This is the extreme position. It is not absolutely necessary to adhere to it. As long as your vision is blurred, this great step toward withdrawal is accomplished. This indrawing of the sense of sight is part of the correct meditation posture.

If you have anything wrong with your eyes or are in any doubt at all as to the advisability of focusing your eyes in close, by all means see your physician and take his advice about practicing this particular part of the total meditation process.

Mantra Yoga

Mantra Yoga is a wonderful form of mental (Raja) Yoga. It is a kind of Yoga of especially practical use for Americans. It is meditation with an object. In this case the object is a sound, word, phrase or worded concept.

Mantra Yoga is the controlling of the mind by repeating to yourself (silently or aloud) a sound, word, phrase or worded concept. It is a vital, challenging and fulfilling venture into the all-important realm of self-knowledge.

In this book you will be told about two Mantras, the two most commonly used and highly esteemed Mantras of the country of India. These Mantras are no more exclusively Indian than the electric light is exclusively American simply because it happened to originate in this country. These two Mantras, like all authentic Yoga Mantras, are universal. They produce the same results for anyone who practices them anywhere in the world.

If the meaning of the sounds or words of a Mantra suggests a different rhythmic pattern from the one prescribed for saying them it is my opinion that the correct saying of them would be of more importance for you.

This is because:

1. When you practice saying a Mantra to yourself, you should coordinate it with your breathing. You will be instructed how to do this as you are taught each Mantra.

By *correctly* coordinating your saying of the Mantra with your breathing, you automatically slow down your breathing. The slower you breathe, the longer you live and the calmer and more composed and tranquil are your nerves and metabolism.

Because you employ the Yogic COMPLETE BREATH, as taught in this book or by any qualified teacher, you also gain physical benefits at the same time, such as purification of the blood, increased energy and vitality. (See COMPLETE BREATH.)

2. The repeating of the Mantra focuses your mind upon one point. This frees you for the duration of your practice from the usual thoughts that go through your mind all day. We will have much to say about thoughts under *The Nature of the Mind.* Your mind becomes quieter and more controlled merely with practice.

3. The thinking or holding in any way in your mind the meaning of the Mantra is pleasant, positive and rewarding if you enjoy so doing. Whenever you wish to engage in this practice, by all means do so to your heart's content. But know that a mental concept such as the meaning of words is but an additional and much denser object in your mind. Eventually a stage is reached where objects as such become an obstruction to the controlling, quieting and stilling of the mind which you desire in your period of meditation. If you have the choice, I would recommend your not worrying about the meaning of the Mantra. The effect of its meaning will occur in any case. Rather attend in the beginning to the correct breathing while practicing Mantra Yoga.

Mantra Yoga is not self-hypnosis or auto-suggestion. On the contrary, it is the path to awakening from the universal hypnotic conditioning to which human beings are subjected.

Mantra Yoga is a mild exercise. You need never worry about

overdoing it. The more you practice it, the better off you are in terms of physical and mental health.

Meditation Technique No. 2: So-Hum

Here is a supremely efficient, practical and profound Mantra.

When you breathe *in* say to yourself (silently) the Sanskrit word *So*.

When you breathe out say the word *Hum*.

Be sure each breath is a COMPLETE BREATH. This will ensure your breaths being long, slow and complete. The correct slowness and completeness of breathing will come automatically after a little practice with this Mantra.

This is a passive meditation technique to be practiced formally when sitting as instructed. It is also an active technique which you can use on many occasions in the midst of everyday life. You can practice So-Hum while walking, waiting, riding from one place to another, even while you are driving a car.

The word *So* means "I am." The word *Hum* means "That." (See *What is Peace?*)

The Benefits of Practicing So-Hum:

1. This Mantra regulates your breathing in a way that results in the greatest health to your body.

2. It calms the nerves.

3. It calms and quiets the mind.

4. It produces, with practice, control over your mind.

5. It produces an alertness, cool-headedness, poise, composure and greater general mental awareness.

The Nature of the Mind

When one speaks of "The Nature of the Mind" the listener might be inclined to say, "What audacity! Whole books of psychology have barely touched the surface of that vast subject." The Yogi answers that Western psychology at its best sees a few of the trees but has never yet had a view of the forest, its size, shape, location and full dimension. Modern psychology paints a very complex picture of the mind and would label many of the Yogis' statements about the mind as being oversimplified.

But complexity has nothing to do with depth or closeness to the truth. Indeed, the greatest truths have a simplicity that is hard for our complexity-oriented minds to grasp.

We have already said two things about the mind that might have come as new concepts to you. One was that the mind has a substance, that it is made of something. The other was that the substance of which the mind is made is forever moving, vibrating restlessly and ceaselessly.

Remembering that what we refer to as "mind" is the conscious and subconscious mind that is functioning at this very moment and throughout your everyday life, we will now further describe the Yogis' viewpoint on the matter in plain, down-to-earth terms.

1. The Yogis thoroughly advise against worshiping the mind.

The everyday mind and its chief claim to authority, namely "logic," is revered far too highly by man. We are indoctrinated to look to the mind as the great solver of problems and our most competent guide through life. We also tend to be awed by the so-called great achievements of the logical intellect. Once you know its true nature, it becomes plain that it does not deserve adulation.

2. The everyday mind—conscious and subconscious—is a machine.

Yes, the mind is a machine, a mechanism and nothing more. That which gives us the impression of being the source of intelligence, consciousness and insight is a mechanical apparatus, a super-computer and data selector.

Intelligence or consciousness comes from a source other than the apparatus that is our everyday, logical mind.

This machine is very much like a robot that, because it functions so well, has come to think of itself as a qualified self-governing entity. The mind is like a servant who has taken over the household of his master. He has so convinced the master that he and he alone knows best and can do best that the master, in relinquishing little by little his original authority, has come to forget entirely that the servant—in this case the mind—has ever been in any other capacity.

You are the actual master. Your mind is actually your servant and tool. Yet you have come to be dependent on its ways, caprices, opinions, guidance, theories, conclusions, etc. This servant who takes over the household of the master lives and is obsessed by one principle: self-preservation. The mind knows that, once the master awakens to the true situation and reassumes his original authority, its power is gone. The mind is alert every second of the day and night to make certain that this never happens.

3. The mind is treacherous.

The everyday mind, this so-called rational "intellectual" mind, is untrustworthy so long as it is in the position of master.

All its guidance, advice, leadership and problem-solving is aimed at producing more "problems" to be solved. Its trick is to always have problems (which you are under the impression are *your* problems), the solution of which is always soon to be arrived at or later to be arrived at if you adhere to the "plan," usually quite logical and reasonable, that your mind has arranged to be the right path for you to follow. We spend years coping with and solving problems that didn't exist or never were problems to begin with.

4. Most thoughts are worthless.

If you will observe the thoughts that come and go through your conscious mind throughout the day, you will note the useless, wasteful and, to a considerable extent, trashy nature of them. Daydreams are nearly always absurd and out of touch with reality. You keep up a running dialogue with yourself that serves no purpose whatever, save to throw those precious minutes and hours of your life away. All through the day your mind lusts after or dreams of what it cannot have or what it is not about to actually go about getting. It gossips, comes to wrong conclusions and much of the time engages in thoughts that are unworthy of a human being whose spark of life is forever burning to its end. Your mind, in its uncontrolled, wayward flight, does everything from cajoling, flattering and puffing up a false ego in you to crushing you with unnecessary, baseless guilt and self-recrimination. It will sink to any depth of degradation to keep itself and you from realizing for a moment that it has not the vaguest connection with reality.

5. The mind is the source of illusions.

The world is known by the knower in us after it has been filtered through our everyday mind (the calculating machine). This is like seeing things only through colored lenses. All is colored by the lens. All is censored and distorted by our minds.

You are not your mind. Your mind is not you. Your mind is no more you than your arm or head is. It is a wonderful, vital part of you but of no greater importance than any other organ or system in your make-up. But from early childhood this mental apparatus has contrived to make us identify ourselves with it.

Your mind does not necessarily know what is best for you. The illusion it propagates is that it and it alone is best equipped to give you the proper advice in all situations. In truth it is not at all an efficient and dependable guide.

It is not the source of pure intelligence or consciousness.

It is not looking out for your best interests.

The function of Raja Yoga is to control this runaway everyday mind. By so doing, you will see it for what it is, and you will verify the foregoing statements regarding it. When you relegate your mind to its proper place as your tool, you will ultimately see who and what is the "you" that this mind has been plaguing you about since your earliest memory.

Your relationship with your mind before gaining control over it is like a person born and raised in a room with a television set playing loudly. He does not know that he is able and supposed to turn the machine off when he doesn't feel like hearing the same old programs over again. Indeed, he does not know how to turn the machine off and rest himself from its empty tyranny.

The need for gaining control of the mind is uppermost. The

intellectual mind is the cause of every dissension, and it is the waster of your life.

The everyday mind, with its thoughts, its logic, its reason, its eternal thinking "about" things and "about" life, its rehashing of the dead past, its fantasies of the future, is *the* obstruction to man's realization of who and what he really is. Your everyday mind is your chief bondage.

Mental Technique No. 3: Om

OM is considered in India to be the highest or prime Mantra. It is said to be, when performed correctly, the sound of the totality of the manifested universe.

OM is, in my opinion, a less practical Mantra for Americans because of the difficulty of practicing it as frequently and in as many circumstances as SO-HUM.

I recommend it as a passive (sitting) meditation technique to be practiced when you are alone.

Practice it aloud. Take a COMPLETE BREATH. The exhalation of the COMPLETE BREATH occurs simultaneously with the saying of the sound OM. Make the sound as long as your outgoing breath. Start the sound—the sound of the "O"—low in your organism, near the navel region where the expulsion of your COMPLETE BREATH begins. It should end with a long resonance—the sound of the "m"—that feels as if it were emanating from or resonating through the head.

OM is quieting for the mind, clearing it of wasteful content. It calms the nerves and metabolism, and when practiced sincerely along with your other physical and mental techniques produces insight into the nature of your self.

Yoga and Metaphysics, the Occult and ESP

To those who enter the field of mind control, there are two paths open. One is the path of Yoga, or spiritual liberation. The other is the path of power.

The path of power is metaphysics. Metaphysics is the controlling of the circumstances and matter of the world around us by means of concentrated mind control.

Through the science of metaphysics one may learn how to win friends and influence people, attain greater business, professional or political success, become rich and powerful, etc. But by this means one does not and cannot attain peace or wisdom. Metaphysics never liberates your true nature from the hands of ever-renewed suffering. In fact, the use of any power is a dire backward step on the road to enlightenment.

Occultism consists of all those studies which develop the so-called supernatural powers such as "astral" projection, clairvoyance and telepathic communication. Persons involving themselves with these subjects range from the curious to those who are pathologically superstitious through those whose personal insecurity is so great that these studies are their one claim to "special" accomplishment.

To the true Yogi, metaphysical achievement and occultism are both looked upon with abhorrence. When held before the light of the true goal of man's life on earth, they seem vain and meaningless enterprises, deadly to spiritual growth. The Yogi advises: Shun power and shun all paths to power.

As to extrasensory perception (ESP), the Yogis have known of this for centuries. The present research on ESP is on a rudimentary level to the Yogis. If a person practices Yoga seriously and correctly over a sufficient period of time, he can stimulate and develop certain parts of his psychic makeup which in nearly all people lie dormant throughout life. This includes extrasensory perception. The development of these dormant but natural abilities in man is a *by-product* of Yoga. It must not be sought after. He *who strives after or seeks* any psychic power, even the simplest extrasensory perception, moves backward on the path to true and lasting peace and self-knowledge. If you would be a sincere and genuine student of Yoga, you must once and forever cast aside metaphysics, the hocus-pocus of occultism and the *desire* to attain ESP.

Mental Technique No. 4: Meditation on the Breath

MEDITATION ON THE BREATH is one of the oldest and most widely used meditative practices.

It consists of first sitting still in the meditation posture, with your breath already established in a long, slow, quiet rhythm by the correct practice of ALTERNATE NOSTRIL BREATHING. You then place your mind—your entire attention—upon the breath as it enters, moves within and leaves your body.

At first it is sufficient to follow the course of each breath from the time it enters to the time it leaves your body.

Later you should attempt to keep your mind on that place where the air leaves the great ocean of air around you and is drawn into your body and on that place where the current of breath, upon leaving your body, merges once again with the atmosphere.

Observe your breath. That is the first step. Do not allow your mind to leave the point of attention, to wander anywhere.

Any time your mind has wandered during meditation and you suddenly find that you have been back in the midst of daily life again, reliving the old clashes and situations of the day or dreaming again the old fruitless daydreams, never scold yourself. Berating yourself is a backward step. *Do not react at all.* Simply bring your mind back to the point of concentration and continue meditating. Why feel angry or bad about a poor machine that has been used to having its own way for the length of your entire life?

Another thing to remember is *never to close your eyes during meditation.* Lower your lids but do not close your eyes. You should always *be able* to see the small circle in which you are seated, although your attention will be on the point of meditation. If you close your eyes during meditation, you are practicing incorrectly. Sleepiness is often the result of closing the eyes during meditation. Sloth is invariably the result.

MEDITATION ON THE BREATH may seem ridiculously simple to you, considering the results claimed for the Raja Yoga techniques. But that view is dispelled after you practice it for a time.

Once experiencing the profound clarifying, stabilizing and quieting effect upon your mind of this meditation technique, you will no longer allow your intellect to appraise it from the point of view of an outsider.

The breath controls the mind. As the breath functions, so functions your mind. If your breath is short and wavering, your mind will be erratic and nervous. If your breath is long, even and complete your mind will be calm, controlled and lucid.

By practicing this present meditation technique, you will know this as a fact of experience. You will also come to learn other facts concerning yourself, the depth of which you will realize at once. (One thing which might come as a rather amazing new realization to you is the fact that you are not doing any breathing at all but that you are being breathed.)

As you can see by now, one of the first functions of meditation or mind control is for the student to establish control over the *thoughts* that go through his or her mind. The Yogi is not interested in substituting so-called good or positive thoughts for so-called bad or negative thoughts. The true, lasting and real peace which Yoga gives is far beyond whether a thought is positive or negative. The Yogi seeks the ability to shut off the interior "television set" entirely at will. With correct practice he attains it.

The techniques you have learned all contribute to your accomplishing this end. Proper use of your breath is the key.

In order to control your thoughts, it is necessary to first slow down their pace. Conscious thoughts are the prime weapon of the mechanical mind. By correct Yogic meditation and breathing, you do slow the pace in which thoughts enter, go through their performance and leave the mind.

You may say, "But they come rushing in and out of my mind from who knows where. There is such a never-ending quantity of them. How can I control such an army of thoughts, especially considering the renewed vigor with which they come once I start trying to control them?"

The answer is: do not be deceived by the supposedly great amount of thoughts that come into your consciousness. For one thing, the variety is not as vast as you imagine. The same thoughts really do repeat themselves over and over again through each day with very little variation.

Another factor is that only one thought can occupy your mind —your conscious attention—at one time. This simplifies the task of mind control. It is like fighting an army but being able to ambush one soldier of it at a time.

Therefore, correct Yogic breathing calms and slows down the frantic, agitated pace of your mind. Meditation (using any authentic Yogic technique, so long as it is practiced correctly) enables you in time to be free of the tyranny of the uncontrolled parade of thoughts. Controlling and stilling the movements of the mind will reveal to you your true self. Once knowing your real self, you will attain the peace that is forever beyond the analysis and understanding of this intellectual mechanical mind in which you are now trapped.

Mental Technique No. 5: Meditation Without an Object

MEDITATION WITHOUT AN OBJECT is the step beyond MEDITATION ON THE BREATH. It consists of sitting as for all passive meditation—after correct preparation—and not allowing thoughts to enter your mind. Only practice can teach you this skill.

You should practice the other meditation technique given in this book in order to know what you are doing and to guarantee the most efficient progress. I recommend practicing each mental technique for one full week in the order in which they are presented in this book. Then you may use whichever one of these suits your particular nature.

This meditation is indeed the highest adventure available or ever known to man. It is the journey to that Shangrila which resides lost and nearly forgotten within each of us. Yet the end of this journey is closer to you than your own breath.

In this journey into yourself, the technique of meditation on your breath becomes a comfortable and ever-convenient camp to which you can return at any time.

There is no time limit on the practice of this meditation. You must only suit the amount of time you practice pure, or objectless, meditation to your way of life. Never bypass any of your everyday responsibilities in order to meditate. Find your time to practice Raja Yoga only if you have met or know that you will meet the obligations of your daily life.

Morning, when it is quiet, is the best time to practice Raja Yoga. Sunset is a splendid time. But do not enslave yourself to unnecessary rituals. Any time you meditate is a good time.

Active Meditation

Active meditation consists of those mental techniques that are performed in the midst of the action of everyday life.

When walking. It is better to observe yourself than to day-dream. You are real; dreams are false and shallow.

When walking you can practice the COMPLETE BREATH. You can also practice the Mantra "So-Hum." A lifetime of dreaming or living in the imagination is a total waste. (By the word "dreaming" we do not mean practical short- or long-range planning nor do we refer to the creative visioning of an artist.) How incalculable, then, is the value of a meditative practice which makes you all the more alive and aware.

An old Japanese Yogic proverb says: "When walking, pay attention to your feet." Childish? Absurdly simple? Try it and see the results. See the immediate difference in your bearing, composure and tranquility.

Allowing the everyday mind to indulge itself in its opiate of dreams leaves life unfruitful and unfulfilled and in the end unlived. Self-observation reveals you to yourself and builds the strength of character that comes with acts of self-discipline.

When waiting. The act of waiting is a fine time to practice your favorite meditation technique. The very fact that you are in a situation which is demanding upon your patience makes the occasion of greater interest. For one thing, you will see for yourself the ability of Yoga to change an irritating or at least what is usually a non-productive period of time into one of vital importance and accomplishment.

Once again start with breathing. Do not make any motions that will possibly draw any attention to you. After establishing your breathing correctly, you can practice Mantra Yoga (So-Hum) or meditate upon your breath.

Simply be a little less formal about it since you are out in everyday life. You need not focus your eyes inward to the extent you would in the privacy of your home. Keep any bodily movements restrained and unnoticeable.

By so practicing Yoga in the midst of life, you transform what would otherwise be time wasted into a time of developing and fulfilling your physical, mental and spiritual faculties.

When driving. Many Americans spend an hour a day or more driving an automobile. In a quiet, anonymous way you can use this time to practice breathing and certain mental techniques. Modify all techniques so that they cannot be seen or interfere with the acts you must perform.

By applying even this time of driving a car—and it is not uncommon at all to drive for twenty or more minutes at a time— to Yoga, you will profit greatly. When you arrive at your destination you will not only be untouched by the usual irritations of traffic, but you will be refreshed, calmed and fortified.

When working. If your occupation is mechanical, instead of "talking to yourself" you could not do better than to practice a Mantra or Yogic breathing or another mental technique that suits you in such circumstances.

These suggestions regarding active meditation have touched upon what is indeed a wonderful subject. You can go through life, from the marketplace to the executive's office, perform your daily work with efficiency and cheerfulness, while unknown to all save yourself you are engaged in the profoundest mental and spiritual exercises known to man.

The notion that a true Yogi must retire to a mountain-top retreat applies only to those whose nature would have led them to a solitary way of life whether they practiced Yoga or not. Going to the hills or to a retreat of equivalent solitude is a delightful temporary prospect for the average person if the opportunity happens to arise. But the sincere student of Yoga will practice wherever he is.

As you walk the streets of life, your everyday mind will never cease striving to cheat you out of living. It will ply you with fantasies, arguments, doubts, desires, absurd memories which it ever tempts you to relive, and other wastes of this, your priceless moment of eternity. Keep in mind that the *mere remembering of Yoga,* the mere bringing to mind of the Raja Yoga techniques that you know, is an actual step of meditation.

Do not believe anything that anyone says about Raja Yoga. It is more important for you to put it to the test of practice. Then see the difference between living like a leaf blown before every wind of mental desire, anxiety and strife and living as the vital soul you are, the living manifestation of an immortal spirit.

Review of Raja Yoga Principles

Body and mind are one thing. They are but two sides of one organism. What happens to one happens to the other. In Hatha Yoga we use the body to develop and perfect both body and mind. In Raja Yoga we work directly with the mind.

The breath is essential in all Yoga. Proper use of the breath increases bodily health, purifies the blood and calms and strengthens the nervous system. The breath also directly affects the mind.

In Yoga we use the breath to quiet and control the mind. The mental techniques of Raja Yoga or correct meditation, aim at stilling the restlessness and ceaseless moving of the mind-substance.

Once the mind is controlled in this way, real peace is experienced.

What Is Peace?

Peace is not a trance nor any trancelike state. The still posture of formal meditation is a part of the means for attaining the peace about which the Yogi speaks.

Dreams have no place in Yoga. Indeed, Yoga is altogether against substituting dreams or imagination for reality or the moment of living. The Yoga way is to know what you are doing at all times, to be self-possessed. Yoga is the practice of mindfulness of the living moment.

Neither is real peace that anemic world of positive thinking where "negative" thoughts have been replaced by "positive" thoughts. Yes, one can certainly achieve cheerfulness, good will, an increase of what some consider to be "happiness" and perhaps worldly success by means of positive thinking. But none of these have the slightest thing to do with peace.

Peace is an experience. It is an experience that has the directness of the experience of touch. But not even the simplest sense experience can intimate the clarity or sureness or reality of the experience of actual peace. The experience of peace has more certainty than the very knowledge that you exist.

Peace is the direct experience-knowledge of who you are. When the bonds of the delusive and insatiable appetite of your senses are broken, when the distractions of your mind are overcome, when you have transcended the wasteful imagination of your mind by controlling it, then does the everyday mind, like a plant uprooted, die.

This is what is meant by dying in order to live. For when the tyranny of this false mind is overthrown, the mind dies. When it dies, it disappears. And when it disappears, there in its place, after all the waiting and all the endless ups and downs of earthly suffering, is the real mind.

The real mind is unbounded. It has no beginning and no end. It is not born nor does it die. It has no form. It has no name. It is beyond all qualities. It is the source and eternal maintainer of all existence.

It has been called by many names: Universal Mind, the Absolute, Tao, the Brahman and numerous others. It does not matter what anyone calls it. All names are but labels used in an attempt to communicate.

The Universal Mind cannot be described. It can only be experienced. It is beyond the scope of the everyday mind—this mechanical, intellectual, so-called logical mind mechanism. In fact, as previously stated, the everyday mind, with all its logic and reason, with its movement and imaginings, is the ultimate obstruction to your experiencing Universal Mind.

Once experiencing Universal Mind, you know for all time who you are. You are Universal Mind. You are That. You have never been anything else and never can be anything else. You are Universal Mind at this very moment, now and forever. Only you and your realization of this one irrefutable fact of life are cloaked by the illusions of your everyday mind.

You will know the network of illusions with which your everyday mind veils you from your true self. It tells you that you are your body. It tells you that you are your mind. It incites you to desire and to strive to "satisfy" your senses.

It uses every device to keep you away from your realization, your experience of your true and eternal self.

But of all its tricks and deceptions, of all its desperate lies, there is one notion that has been implanted deep in the recesses of every human being which is the primary illusion that veils us from our true nature. This is the notion that you are a separate individual being, a separated entity, a personality, an "I."

As Gautama Buddha said:

". . . no (Yogi) who is a real (Yogi) cherishes the idea of an ego-entity, a personality, a being, or a separated individuality."

All things—mind, body, matter and force—are but forms of and in Universal Mind, the great Self which is your only real identity.

In the moment of enlightenment that which you now know as your self, that which you now call "I," is not so much shed as a snake casts off the old skin or as life sheds itself of a physical body; rather, it merges into Universal Mind like a "dewdrop merging into the shining sea." The part becomes the whole. That is fulfillment.

Conclusion

You can go as far as you want with Yoga. The entire path is open to you. How far you go depends only on yourself, your needs, your interest, your predispositions.

You should, however, use Raja Yoga for the practical benefits it brings. We all need to calm our nerves and quiet our minds. Do not think of the results of practicing meditation, especially the ultimate spiritual results. Practice meditation for the immediate improvement and satisfaction it brings; this assures the best results.

You do not have to attain realization of Universal Mind in order to profit from this ancient science. Simple everyday practice will reap results for you of greater value than you can now calculate. Meditation increases poise, calmness of body, emotions and mind, mental clarity, self-control, inner peace and strength of character.

Do not talk about Raja Yoga or your practice of meditation to anyone. Talking about it greatly decreases a person's ability to practice it. Once you begin to feel the wonderful change toward peace and stability that comes with systematic meditation, be especially careful of taking any pride in your study or practice of Yoga. Spiritual pride is certain death. A sign of a true Yogi is humility, especially regarding Yoga.

Raja Yoga is for use in this life in this world. You will come out of any correctly practiced interval of meditation fortified, strengthened, more alive and better able to function creatively or at the mechanical tasks of everyday life.

Unless stated specifically in the description of each mental technique, there is no time limit on the practice of meditation. Never neglect important duties and worldly responsibilities to prolong your meditation. But plan your time carefully to fit sufficient Yoga practice into your daily life so that you are free from conflict.

Always remember this cardinal principle of Yoga as stated by the most ancient and authoritative sources and known to be true through thousands of years of practice. There is no *Raja Yoga without Hatha Yoga.* You cannot abuse your body—the house of the spirit—or abandon it by neglect to the destructive influences of the world and hope to achieve peace of mind. There is no peace for the person whose body is sick, underdeveloped or deteriorated.

Practice meditation at the quietest time of day available to you and in as private and quiet a place as possible. *Always begin your meditation with seven rounds of correctly practiced* ALTERNATE NOSTRIL BREATHING. By so doing, you will prepare your nerves, metabolism and mind for meditation, and you will also establish a strong pattern of correct posture. It is best to bathe or shower before practicing Yoga. Be sure the room you practice in is ventilated for maximum fresh air. The place should be private, clean and neat (uncluttered) if possible. Clothing should be loose for comfort and bodily ventilation. In warm weather you may wear abbreviated garb—shorts, etc.—for such comfort. Never practice meditation on a full stomach. If the environment is quiet enough, it is splendid to practice Raja Yoga after performing your physical techniques.

No one can practice Yoga or meditation or attain health or experience peace for you. Practice Yoga assiduously in quiet composure and with perseverance, and all the results will be yours. It is a methodical science, and the results come to those who adhere to the rules.

APPENDIX ONE:
PRACTICE SCHEDULES

FIRST WEEK

Technique	Start with	Each week add	Until you reach	Repeat
ALTERNATE LEG PULL	10 seconds	5 seconds	60 seconds	3 times each leg
COBRA	10 seconds	5 seconds	30 seconds	
SHOULDER STAND	10 seconds	5 seconds	30 seconds	3 times
HALF LOTUS	3 minutes	15 seconds	5 minutes	1 time
COMPLETE BREATH	See page 62			
CANDLE	See page 100			
CONCENTRATION	3 minutes eyes open. 3 minutes eyes closed.			

SECOND WEEK

Practice the Yoga techniques you did in the first week and then add:

Technique	Start with	Each week add	Until you reach	Repeat
HALF LOCUST	5 seconds each leg	5 seconds	30 seconds	3 times each leg
PLOUGH	5 seconds each position	5 seconds to each position	30 seconds each position	3 times
CLEANSING BREATH	2 rounds of 10 breaths	1 round	6 rounds of 10 breaths	
SO-HUM				

THIRD WEEK

Practice the Yoga techniques you did in the first and second weeks and then add:

Technique	Start with	Each week add	Until you reach	Repeat
ABDOMINAL CONTRACTION	5 sets of 5	(See Abdominal Contraction)	10 sets of 10	
TWIST	10 seconds each side	5 seconds	30 seconds each side	3 times each side
LEG AND BACK STRETCH	10 seconds	5 seconds	60 seconds	3 times
LOCUST	5 seconds	1 second	10 seconds	3 times
OM				

FOURTH WEEK

Practice the techniques you did in the first three weeks and then add:

Technique	Start with	Each week add	Until you reach	Repeat
Bow	5 seconds	1 second	15 seconds	3 times
Lion	10 seconds	5 seconds	30 seconds	3 times
Fish	10 seconds	5 seconds	45 seconds (see Fish posture)	3 times
Neti	This technique is optional, to be used if needed or desired.			
Meditation on the Breath				

Keep a careful record of your time increases for each technique.

FIFTH WEEK

Practice the techniques you have learned so far and then add:

Technique	Start with	Each week add	Until you reach	Repeat
HEAD STAND	15 seconds	15 seconds	5 minutes	once each day
ALTERNATE NOSTRIL BREATHING	7 rounds			See page 14
FULL LOTUS	See page 64			
MEDITATION WITHOUT AN OBJECT				

Sixth Week

At this point divide the techniques you have been practicing into the following three groups.

Group 1

Abdominal Contraction
Cobra
Locust (or Half Locust)
Bow
Fish
Shoulder Stand
Lion
Complete Breath
Alternate Nostril Breathing
Meditation Technique

Group 2

Abdominal Contraction
Alternate Leg Pull
Plough
Leg and Back Stretch
Twist
Shoulder Stand (or Head Stand)
Lion
Cleansing Breath
Alternate Nostril Breathing
Meditation Technique

Group 3

Abdominal Contraction
Shoulder Stand
Lion
Cleansing Breath
Complete Breath
Alternate Nostril Breathing

Practice Group 1 on one day. The next day practice Group 2. On the third day practice Group 3. Then Group 1 again. Then Group 2. Then Group 3, etc.
For example:

Monday	Tuesday	Wednesday	Thursday	Friday	Saturday	Sunday
Group 1	Group 2	Group 3	Group 1	Group 2	Group 3	Group 1

Monday	Tuesday	Wednesday	Thursday	Friday	Saturday	Sunday
Group 2	Group 3	Group 1	Group 2	Group 3	Group 1	Group 2

It becomes an endless cycle, only altered by the time that you add to each technique as the weeks pass.

If you miss a day altogether, then you simply continue with the next group as if your schedule had not been interrupted at all.

Observe Group 3. There are no stretching postures included here (except the highly specialized LION posture). Group 3 has been designed to rest your body from the great stretches.

By resting your body every third day, you are actually helping to speed your progress. If you were to use the stretching postures every day, your body would begin to rebel, and it would stiffen up periodically. This stiffening would be both uncomfortable and demoralizing.

No learning ever proceeds in a straight line. Learning occurs in a series of steps forward alternating with smaller steps backward. Let us say it is like taking three steps forward and one step back, three forward, one back. To practice a full schedule every day would be to break this basic law of learning.

By systematically resting your body from the postures in the manner indicated, you absorb the body's primitive resistance, and your progress in Yoga goes forward smoothly.

APPENDIX TWO:
PROGRAMS FOR
SPECIAL GROUPS

The more of these basic postures and techniques that you can perform each day, the greater will be the benefits to you. But we understand how your time can be taken up by responsibilities.

Therefore, we are recommending here those postures and techniques which most apply to you according to your way of life. This by no means suggests that you eliminate any of the twenty life-giving techniques taught in this book but rather suggests which ones you should *emphasize* more strongly and around which you should build your daily practice schedule.

For the Housewife

Emphasize the SHOULDER STAND, COBRA, LION, ALTERNATE LEG PULL and ALTERNATE NOSTRIL BREATHING. Nerves and fatigue are the housewife's problems. Not too many men realize that the day an industrious housewife puts in could wear out the average man. But at the same time the housewife has access to the home and can arrange things in order to have the half hour necessary to put in a good session of Yoga before being swept up in the chores that occupy the dinner hours.

It is a good idea for the housewife to take as her time for Yoga an interval before her husband comes home from work. Try to arrange a quiet period of time so that you can not only practice Yoga but also take a good rest after it in the peaceful mood that you will be in after your workout.

If you prefer, as many women do, to practice Yoga in the evening, it is good to do the SHOULDER STAND before dinner and to take a five minute rest after doing it.

It is advisable to do the ALTERNATE NOSTRIL BREATHING at a selected quiet interlude shortly before the arrival of the dinner-time activities.

One of the greatest blessings you can bestow upon your children is to teach them the Yoga postures as soon as they are able to learn them. A child usually has enough self-control and understanding to learn these simple techniques at about the age of nine.

For Sedentary Workers

Use the ABDOMINAL CONTRACTION, LION and COMPLETE BREATH *during your working day* if you can get a few minutes of privacy.

If you are one of the millions of persons in the United States who must sit at a desk for eight hours a day or engage for the greater part of the day in that kind of inactivity, you are subject to a physical problem the magnitude of which can hardly be calculated in terms of personal misery or loss of national efficiency. That is the stiffening and contracting of your spine and of the tendons and ligaments of your body. In the light of what you have learned about the human body in the Hatha Yoga section, this brings to mind all the tension and related negative conditions which are caused by this stiffening.

The sedentary worker, besides losing the full use of his body because of its stiffening, in the majority of cases slowly acquires a sunken chest and flabby dropped abdomen. The words "sunken chest" do not signify only those extreme cases in which this condition is noticeable, but apply to the condition of impaired breathing which invariably results from prolonged sitting work.

Sedentary work is an abuse of the body. The toll upon the nervous system through the deformity of the spine due to this work is very great. Breathing is shallow and constricted, resulting in susceptibility to respiratory diseases and also in poor blood quality due to lack of proper oxygenation. Life-force is very deficient, and postural malformities, though subtle at first, exact a terrible price with the passing years.

No man or woman on earth need ever be a bent, tottering old person. Such a tragic condition, which we see around us every day, is only the result of improper care of the body. You have the knowledge now that can enable you to prevent that state from ever being your fate.

People employed in office work or other sedentary occupations are in foremost need of Hatha Yoga. To these people we say: practice your stretching postures faithfully and regularly, and these hazards of your occupation will be eliminated. Once eliminated, they will be prevented from ever returning again. Regular practice of the great stretches you learned in this book will put you in a state of physical well-being that you never dreamed possible. You will have a new-found vitality and alertness. Your work will become much more enjoyable, and you will perform it with much more efficiency.

Practice all the techniques you now know, but emphasize the concave and convex stretches at home.

For Active or Manual Workers

This category comprises a variety of occupations including the many kinds of laborers and salesmen.

The fact that in one's occupation the body is made to move actively does not mean at all that it will be any more limber than the next person's. The movement of the body during everyday work puts into play only certain specific sets of muscles. The active worker may bend, but he does not stretch in a way that gives his or her body any flexibility.

People in these occupations accumulate as much tension as anyone else and must work out these tension points throughout their bodies by the scientific Yogic stretching postures.

Emphasize in your schedule the SHOULDER STAND. Perform the SHOULDER STAND before you do the other postures to get the blood circulation properly into your head and to regulate the circulation in your legs as well as relieve the distended blood vessels in your legs. Then do your stretching postures with the blood circulation thus adjusted.

You will find that if, instead of flopping down on the sofa or taking a nap or collapsing into a chair upon coming home from a hard day's physical work, you take a shower and then get down on the floor at once and begin your Yoga practice, you will replenish your energy—get your "second wind"—in a way that will take you pleasantly through the rest of the day. The concave stretches, the TWIST, the FISH and the SHOULDER STAND will accomplish this for you.

For Students and Young People

Students will find Hatha Yoga to be of incalculable aid in their studies.

The first advice we give any student is to perform the SHOULDER STAND or the HEAD STAND and ALTERNATE NOSTRIL BREATHING *before starting your homework.* The mental alertness and clarity induced by these practices will have very good effects upon the quality of your school work. You will also be able to overcome the dulling fatigue which comes with prolonged studious activity.

As to fatigue, here is a formula which has aided students of all grade levels from fifth grade through college. At about the half-way point in your daily homework routine, get up from your studies and do your Yoga. Never neglect the PLOUGH and the COBRA. For clearing the mind include the CLEANSING BREATH followed by the COMPLETE BREATH.

Take a minute or so to rest after each posture, and then resume your studies. The ten to twenty minutes that it took you to perform your Yoga postures—depending on the stage of practice you are at—will reward you with several hours of tension-free alertness. The positive effects of these techniques are cumulative and last longer as you continue to practice every day.

When we speak of energy, bear in mind that we do not mean a restless kind of energy that might distract you from your study. This energy is a vitality that works through an organism whose metabolism has been regulated and calmed. It gives you endurance.

If you have another time of the day in which you prefer to do your Hatha Yoga postures, that is fine. Nonetheless, we strongly urge you to precede your period of studies with one of the inversion postures—SHOULDER or HEAD STAND—and with the ALTERNATE NOSTRIL BREATHING (at least five rounds done correctly). Whenever you do any conscious breathing techniques, be sure to perform them with the correct bodily movements to make certain that each breath is *complete*.

Experience with numerous students has proved that the practice of Yoga in conjunction with school work results in better scholastic achievement. When you consider that the quality of your work in school, whether elementary school, high school or college, has a direct influence on your life in terms of success, it is plain to see that the few minutes of Yoga you can correctly practice each day may be calculated in thousands of dollars worth of value above and beyond the priceless gift of health.

For Senior Citizens

We have taught people as old as eighty-one. In a year of correct practice remarkable transformations have taken place in every case. We have seen wrinkles disappear, ossified bodies become more limber than the average thirty-five-year-old, vitality and physical endurance return to an astonishing degree, eyes and minds grow bright and sharp once more. These are not exaggerations but proven facts. They attest to the power of Yoga and to its gentleness.

There are certain specific points, however, which must be kept in mind by persons who begin the study of Yoga when already in their later years. Older people must apply themselves to these postures with *much more care and gentleness* than younger persons would.

At the slightest discomfort, stop. Start over from the beginning with infinite gentleness. Don't do anything that pains you. If you have ever had a pathological condition, get the approval of your physician. It has been our experience that most physicians are glad to have older people practice Yoga. You must know that when a Yoga posture hurts, you are doing it wrong or just too strenuously. Patience is the key, not effort.

If you are on in years and especially if you are not in the best condition for your age, be careful in attempting the SHOULDER STAND. Experiment in the most gradual way. Lie on the floor with your legs up against the wall at first. Use the wall for as long as you must. Lie face down on your bed and allow your head to hang down over the side at first to see how your organism reacts to inversion. Senior citizens should *not* practice the HEAD STAND.

For elderly persons, the stretches are more important. *Senility is synonymous with stiffness of the spine.* No matter how old a person is, if the spine is flexible and able to bend to its natural capacity, he or she will never become senile. The spinal cord is the communication line of the body, and all messages to and from the brain must travel through this cord. If the spine is atrophied and stiff, semi-ossified through lifelong poor usage or lack of use, the impulses cannot travel properly to and fro. Certain key functions of the mind deteriorate; memory becomes faulty; sense functioning is impaired. This needless tragedy can be overcome to a very great extent even if its symptoms have begun to appear. It can certainly be prevented. It is only a matter of slowly and systematically bringing back the natural flexibility of the spinal column through the Yogic postures. Improvement of circulation is necessary and comes automatically with this practice.

We recommend that senior citizens first practice the breathing techniques. Next emphasize the stretching postures to recondition the spine. After that experiment with the SHOULDER STAND if you wish. Wait for three months after beginning the stretching techniques before commencing the SHOULDER STAND if it gives you any difficulty at first.

For Entertainers

Here we include a wide variety of professionals—musicians, actors, singers, speakers and other entertainers. Some of the most outstanding personalities in the world of entertainment today are devoted students of Yoga. Yehudi Menuhin, Gloria Swanson, Cary Grant and Olivia de Havilland are but a few from the long list of people in the artistic and entertainment world who know the value of this ancient science. Many of these people were already world-recognized in their field when they began practicing Yoga. They have stated that Yoga added greatly to their ability even then.

Yoga gives balance, poise and the additional self-confidence that comes with these traits. Firmness of body, wholesome complexion (due to improved circulation), endurance, vitality and the ability to stay relaxed in the midst of action come with the practice of Yoga. These qualities contribute very much to an artist's work.

Breath control is of uppermost importance to persons who must face the public on stage or before cameras. It is also an integral part of the work in which most entertainers are engaged. Regarding the overcoming of occupational nervousnses before a performance, nothing known to man can compare with ALTERNATE NOSTRIL BREATHING. Tranquilizing pills, no matter what type, always have negative effects, whether it takes weeks, months or years for these effects to manifest themselves. But ALTERNATE NOSTRIL BREATHING performs the function of tranquilizing the nervous system and at the same time is clarifying for the mind and healthy for the body.

Entertainers are subject to their own special kinds of fatigue. They are known to work long hours when engrossed in a production. If you are in this field, you most certainly owe it to yourself to practice the full Yoga regimen as taught in this book, both to offset your occupational hazards and to improve the traits which add to your artistry.

For Business and Professional Men and Women

Try to arrange a time, no matter how brief, to practice certain techniques during your work day.

The ABDOMINAL CONTRACTION, the LION and the COMPLETE BREATH can usually be fitted in. Before lunch is a good time for a workout that will both soothe tense nerves and overcome fatigue.

If you can get down on the floor somewhere in private, by all means do your SHOULDER STAND and then as many of the stretching postures as you can without losing the quiet, unruffled slow-motion. It is better to do one posture correctly than several of them in a hurried, incorrect manner.

For the Family

The preservation and wholesomeness of the family system

should be an uppermost factor in the life of every human being. That which can bring the members of a family together in closer communication and sharing of the same interest is precious indeed. Yoga does this, and in the most pleasant way imaginable. We have seen, time after time, that when a family practices Yoga together—much like a common hobby—wonderful results in terms of the happiness and well-being of the members occur.

A family can practice the postures alone or together, depending upon which way produces the best results. A beautiful thing transpires when all members of a family are involved in this science of self-development. When practiced by a family Yoga produces a harmony which is profoundly important in a time when so many forces are at work undermining the family structure.

A General Rule of Practice

If you are in such circumstance that you cannot adhere to an exact progressive schedule, or if you do not have access to the practice schedule given in this book, then apply the following simple rule.

When sitting down to practice Yoga, first do the cleansing techniques—ABDOMINAL CONTRACTION, NETI, CLEANSING BREATH. Next do the postures. After that practice the breathing techniques, ending your physical workout with ALTERNATE NOSTRIL BREATHING. Then do your meditation, whichever mental technique you employ.

Observe the sequence: cleansing, stretching, breathing, mental. You go from the gross to the refined. You first care for the more impure parts of your organism. Then you scientifically manipulate the whole of your body. After that you work with your breath, which is the link between body and mind. Finally you deal directly with that seemingly insubstantial part of your organism, the mind. Each of these categories prepares you for the techniques to follow so that they can work at top efficiency for you.

INDEX